"During my visit, the doctor had me blow into a peak flow meter to measure the speed of air I could exhale from my lungs. He took other tests, and at the end of my visit said to me, 'I am happy to tell you, you are 100 percent free of asthma."

Katrina Love Senn, former asthmatic

TABLE OF CONTENTS

Introduction

While the number of asthmatics in the U.S. tripled in the last 30 years, Western medicine's message regarding treatment remains the same: "There is no cure for asthma."

However, asthmatics around the world who are exhausted from their relentless symptoms and tired of Western medicine's dogma are coming to an entirely different conclusion.

My journey to finding a cure for asthma began in a $30 hotel room in Panama City, Panama. My then-boyfriend (now husband), who had lived with asthma since the age of six, was experiencing severe and seemingly worsening asthma symptoms. As a fluke, we searched online for "asthma cures." We found asthmastory.com, a comprehensive website created by Jim Quinlan detailing his journey from near-fatal asthma attack to discovering that his asthma was caused by prolific bacteria that could be and ultimately was cured with antibiotics. Jim had not used his inhaler or any asthma medication in 17 years.

We were hopeful.

Fast-forward four months. We were in David's hometown in Spain. David's asthma symptoms were taking him from a person fond of hiking and biking up mountains to a person who was finding simple daily tasks unbearable.

We went to the doctor.

As David was explaining why he came in, he also mentioned the possibility of his asthma being caused by bacteria. David's doctor did what many Western doctors described within these 14 stories did: she laughed.

David left with a prescription for a pile of drugs.

The drug pile provided a much-needed temporary reprieve, but as many asthmatics and those who love them know, the reprieve is short-lived and the possibility of future suffering under Western medical care is practically a guarantee. A few months later, David went to a homeopath that had cured a childhood friend of asthma.

We were hopeful again.

But two visits and six months later, David believed his asthma was the worst it had ever been. Tasks that no one would consider exertion were triggering asthmatic symptoms in David: making breakfast, taking a three-block walk down the street, cutting a watermelon.

His symptoms showed zero mercy. There were days he required his asthma inhaler a dozen times or more. Getting a full night's sleep was an impossibility.

It scares me to think how dangerously close I was to accepting that David's inability to breathe normally numerous times daily was simply part of our routine, not something that needed immediate and substantial attention. It was after he left to go to work on a particularly asthmatic morning that I thought of the words of a woman I had interviewed for my website, thedeliciousday.com, regarding her journey from drug addict to yogini. I had asked her if there was anything anyone could have done for her in the depths of her addiction. Her response was, "Get me to a doctor."

Finding an Eastern medical doctor in an area of the world that speaks Catalan and Spanish when you speak English fluently and Spanish like a decently smart one-and-a-half-year-old was not easy. Eventually, I found a place in Barcelona that was patient enough to put up with both my questions and my Spanish.

2

As I was searching for doctors, I was also doing the only other thing I thought I could do to help David: looking for others who would be willing to share their stories on how they cured themselves of asthma. Writing about people who have cured themselves of diseases Western medicine claims are not curable is something dear to my heart, and as such, I have written rather extensively on topic on The Delicious Day. I thought that if I could collect enough stories on others who have cured asthma, I could not only help David to find his road to recovery, but I could provide others like David with inspiration for finding theirs.

What I found in preparing this book is something I always suspected: David is not alone in his journey towards curing his asthma — not even close. David, from his small town in Catalonia, is now walking on a path that many around the world are walking with him. David had the courage to start this journey, and like the people described within, he has the conviction to finish it. David's story to recovery, also like all the stories within, is very unique to him with the exception of one commonality among all: he and these people all believe that living a life without suffering with asthma is possible. All the people whose stories are shared within — regardless of the cause of their asthma or the number of years they had it or everything doctors had ever told them — knew there was a life without asthma waiting for them, and they went out and got it.

From that commonality, the stories diverge greatly. Asthma is a condition in which a number of different possible triggers result in an over-reactive airway and subsequent difficulty in breathing. The trigger that causes asthma symptoms in one asthmatic may have no effect on another. As there are endless combinations of physiological, psychological, dietary and lifestyle triggers that can cause asthma symptoms, there are also, as shown within, numerous methods in which to cure it.

3

The Western medical approach to asthma is to prescribe a lifetime of medication to lessen the frequency and severity of asthmatic symptoms. This approach has undoubtedly saved the lives of countless people, but it does nothing to cure or completely eliminate the problem.

That is where the stories of these 14 people come in.

These 14 approaches to healing didn't lessen the frequency or severity of asthmatic symptoms – they completely eliminated them – and not just for hours or days but for months, years and decades.

The cures these people used to arrive at a life without asthma are unique to each individual and involved many things, including lifestyle, diet and exercise changes. Some needed to work with unresolved grief. Others used some very unconventional yet highly effective alternative therapies. Some took days, months or years to cure themselves; one woman I spoke to was cured in 90 minutes.

These people come from four different nations on three different continents. Four are doctors. One is a woman who was cured as a teenager. Another is a mother who cured both her children. Many lived the vast majority of their lives with asthma until they found a cure as adults. Others lived decades without asthma and when suddenly diagnosed set out on a path to find a cure. Some used only one treatment to cure themselves; for others, it was a process of trial and error (and more error). Regardless of their individual journeys, they all arrived at the same destination: a life without the thought of or the need for asthma medication.

David and I have found great hope in hearing the stories of these extraordinary people. May you find the same.

p.s.:

1.   In addition to the 14 people who cured themselves of asthma, I spoke with two women who still rely, at times, on their inhalers and asthma medication. Their stories and approaches I found extremely interesting. One woman, Katherine, has drastically reduced her asthma symptoms via diet and lifestyle changes. The other, Katie, has reduced her asthma symptoms to needing her inhaler, as she said, "about two times" a year. I have included their stories in the back of this book with the story of a woman who significantly reduced the asthma symptoms of her son, as I feel the information they provide is invaluable. Their stories are the last three in this collection.

2.   And lastly, the required legal note: the stories within are not intended or implied to be a substitute for professional advice, diagnosis or treatment.

Now on to these 14 extraordinary people…

#1 Cured Her Two Children of Asthma with Vitamin C

At the age of two, Jennifer's daughter was diagnosed with asthma. Then, when her son was only one month old, he was diagnosed as well. Terrified of what the asthma medication was doing to her children's very young bodies, Jennifer and her husband did extensive research to find ways to mitigate the side effects of these drugs. Eight months later, through the administration of elevated doses of vitamin C, Jennifer and her husband not only mitigated the side effects of the asthma medication, but had cured both their children of asthma.

Here is a bit of Jennifer's story.

How did you come to think that vitamin C could help your children?

A friend gave me an allergy book written in 1972. It had a whole chapter on asthma. When I was reading it in 1993 or 1994, the exact same asthma medication was still being prescribed that was being prescribed for asthmatics in 1972. More than anything, I was looking for something to eliminate the side effects of the asthma medication. My kids were not anywhere close to being developed and here I was putting this junk in their bodies and this allergy book — I wish I had the title of it — stated that taking vitamin C in elevated doses would counteract the ill effects of the medicine and lessen the exacerbations from asthma, if not eliminate them. I said, "OK!" I went out and bought a huge bottle of vitamin C and starting giving it to my kids. My son drank a container of powdered formula every other day. He got 500 milligrams of vitamin C in every bottle. To this day, at the first sign of a cold or when feeling sick, my kids will start on vitamin C heavy-duty, and they don't get sick.

Do you have any thoughts on what an "elevated" dosage of vitamin C would be for an adult?

We have done a lot of research on Linus Pauling. Pauling did extensive research on the many benefits of vitamins in improving health and chronic disease. There is also a guy in the Midwest who has done extensive research because his son is schizophrenic. His son takes something like 25,000 milligrams of vitamin C per day. If you tell Western-medicine doctors that you take more than 250 milligrams per day, they flip out because they say you are going to get kidney stones. They say your body can't digest it. I take 5,000 milligrams of vitamin C per day, and I have no problems. I am healthy as a horse and do not get sick. Humans are the only creatures on the planet that do not reproduce our own vitamin C. I worked myself up to 5,000 milligrams a few years ago.

What do you mean by "worked yourself up to"?

You have to work yourself up to it. You can't just take 5,000 milligrams of vitamin C. If you take 5,000 milligrams of vitamin C without working your body up to it, you are going to have violent diarrhea because vitamin C cleans your system. So you start at 500 milligrams, and then each day you take 500 milligrams more. You need to build up your body's acceptance of it. If you talk to doctors who practice orthomolecular treatment, they will tell you how to do it. If you look up vitamin C therapy, you can also learn how to do it. A naturopathic doctor will also tell you how to build up vitamin C levels. There are people who believe you can take anywhere between 15,000 and 50,000 milligrams of vitamin C per day. My medical doctor told me not to take more than 250 milligrams per day. He said to me, "Did you know if you took that much vitamin C in one day that chemotherapy would not work?" And I said, "Of course it would not work, because vitamin C would flush the poison out of you and chemotherapy is poison." There are people who think that vitamin C can cure cancer. There is so much information out there, but because we follow Western medicine, pharmaceuticals and insurance companies, we do not have the studies on what is cheap and natural. It is simply not applied in Western medicine.

Do you have any thoughts on why both of your children had asthma?

If you would have asked me 18 years ago, I wouldn't have known where to begin. Looking back now I have some ideas. My husband has sinus disease and he had horrible allergies. We thought our children's asthma was allergy-related in the beginning. Through the years, we have learned and researched a lot. I do believe asthma is misdiagnosed sometimes. We were able to eliminate all asthmatic symptoms from my daughter only to find out she had sinus disease. My son was completely cured and he is the one that had the worst problems. He was able to cure quicker than my daughter.

Do you believe your daughter ever had asthma or do you believe she was completely misdiagnosed?

I believe she was having asthmatic symptoms due to the fact that her body did not have a filter. She had no sinuses. We did not know that until she was 14 and had a CAT scan and we learned she had only 20 percent of her [total] sinuses. We were able to stop all of her asthmatic exacerbations with vitamin C. She had her first asthma attack at two. We thought it was an allergy problem, but the attacks continued to happen. She was never on steroids. She just needed the nebulizer. It did not happen every day. Her asthma symptoms were more seasonally.

There were days or weeks or months where she did not have any asthmatic symptoms?

Exactly. And then boom, she was down.

What was the Western medicine-prescribed treatment for your daughter?

My daughter was prescribed a nebulizer with a mixture of saline, cromulin sodium and albuterol. She was on that every four hours or as needed. It was not severe. If it was, it would have been more often. Originally, I pursued chiropractors for her and the chiropractor would adjust her and then use a heat lamp on her to loosen up the lungs. The heat lamp was effective, but I did not find going to the chiropractor effective. I continued with heat when she was on the asthma medication. This was before my son came along. Then it became really scary because my son could not breathe as an infant, and that is when my husband and I really went crazy to find out what was going on. We ripped out all the carpeting. We removed all the window treatments. Any fabric we could remove from our house, we removed. Every night, when I went to bed, I had four rags on my nightstand. When I woke up in the morning, I would wash down the entire house before I got them out of bed — all the furniture, floors, walls, everything.

What was the medication prescribed to your son?

He was on saline, cromulin sodium and albuterol plus prednisone, and that is what really snapped me, because I was putting this junk into this infant's mouth. That is when I got crazy about research.

Do you believe cleaning the house every day and removing all the fabrics helped?

We installed a CentralVac. We didn't know what was triggering the attacks. We did not know if it was their bodies or a pollutant, so we eliminated all pollutants. We had the house as clean as it could be, and my son just continued to get worse. I was literally running into the hospital and the pediatricians' offices because they would exacerbate so badly.

What does vitamin C do for asthma?

It totally and completely cleans toxins out of your body, and I can tell you my son has never, ever, ever had another asthma attack. When I brought my son in for his yearly wellness exam, the doctor looked at me and said, "I have not seen you in a year. I made a bet I would see you and admit one of these kids to the hospital based on what you were doing with vitamin C." I told him, "You better start telling your patients about vitamin C." He said to me, "I don't believe it. They must have outgrown the asthma." And I said, "Outgrown what we went through last year?!" He looked at me and said, "Maybe not."

What about side effects of taking elevated doses of vitamin C?

None. I have not seen one whatsoever.

Was vitamin C the only solution for curing your children's asthma, or did you try any other alternative therapies?

I didn't have to. Vitamin C did it. I absolutely 100 percent believe it did it. This guy in the Midwest who studies vitamin C therapy doesn't believe that the amount my kids were taking was enough to cure them, and even he was surprised. My son was getting 8,000 milligrams a day. He said, "There is no way 8,000 milligrams cured it." And I said, "Well, he has never had a problem since." He believes you had to have a minimum of 10,000 per day.

How many milligrams of vitamin C per day was your daughter taking when she had asthma?

My daughter was taking a minimum of 2,000 milligrams per day.

I am curious as to why you sought out a chiropractor.

I did it because it was natural and did not involve chemicals.

But you did not see a positive impact with the chiropractor?

The positive impact was the heat he applied, and I did that at home.

How did you apply heat at home?

I had my daughter lay on a heating pad that was under her chest, and then I would absolutely pound on her back to get her to loosen up what was in her lungs. I timed it and watched the temperature because she was little. I would do it for 15 minutes and then pound on her.

When you say "pound on her," what does that mean?

[Laughing] We taught her to sing while we did it so it would sound funny and seem like a game. But we would literally pat her back very strongly. A kid would be coughing or choking to get what was in their lungs moving. We would do that after every heat treatment and after every treatment with the nebulizer.

Were you doing the heat treatment with your son as well?

Using heat with my son was difficult as he was an infant. He was always warm. We didn't want to increase his body temperature, so we used it very little with him.

You were doing all this 20-ish years ago. Do you believe anything has changed since then regarding how asthma is treated by Western medicine?

Nope. It has stayed exactly the same, while I'm jumping up and down saying, "Start pumping the vitamin C." Nothing has changed. Same medications, same treatments — everything is exactly the same. I also believe the diagnosis is easy for doctors — children need more attention to find out what is really happening. We also need to make sure we are simply not treating with drugs. Alternatives are out there.

My kids don't have asthma anymore, and they were diagnosed with asthma by Western medical doctors. My daughter was hospitalized three times with asthma and my son was hospitalized once. They were on all the medications. We went through the whole circus. My kids had asthma and now they don't have asthma. You can judge it for yourself, but I watched it happen. My husband and I made it happen. We got as much information as we could, and we did it. The medication they give you does not cure asthma. It treats it. What did we do differently? One thing: we administered vitamin C in high doses. They are not on medication anymore, and never were again.

This all happened and they were both cured in eight months?

Yes. We did not stop giving them vitamin C after they were cured. As my son got older and started chewing his food, I lightened it to 2,000 milligrams. I was handing vitamin C out like candy. Once you build up the vitamin C in your body, you will see a lessening of exacerbations. I swear you will see it.

Anything else you would like to add?

You need to drink a lot of water if you are going to take lots of vitamin C. Vitamin C tends to dehydrate, because it is doing its job. You need the fluids to replenish what you flush out. You do not need to drink gallons and gallons, but you need to stay hydrated. I drink three liters of water every day plus whatever else I drink. Find your balance.

...

#2 Cured Her Asthma in 90 Minutes

Jeanette Chasworth suffered many bouts of bronchitis as a child, but was not diagnosed with asthma until her early 20s. For four years after Jeanette was diagnosed, she looked unsuccessfully for a cure. A chance meeting between her father and a healer would turn Jeanette's life and health around. After one 90-minute session with this healer, Jeanette has never had to use her inhaler or asthma medication again. That was over 16 years ago.

Here is a bit of her story.

What were the approaches you tried to cure your asthma?

I went to doctors and they could not offer anything that helped. I tried swimming, which was really helpful. Doctors gave me inhalers. They also gave me this pill and other medication and I ended up with a bloody nose and had to go to the hospital because of it. I did all kinds of inhalers and medication, but they were not helping me. They were helping me so I could breathe, but they were not getting me to a point where I did not need them, or where I even felt good. You have all of those drugs in you, and you just feel icky.

Whenever I got stressed out, I would have an asthma attack. My dad happened across a guy who said he could cure me. At that point, I would have done just about anything to breathe again. He called himself a metaphysical healer. I did not know what to expect. My parents said he was a little unorthodox, but he said he could heal me, so I was game.

What happened in your visit with him?

He did muscle testing. He explained to me that every organ is associated with an emotion. The lungs are associated with depression. As he was doing muscle testing he was telling me things about myself and all I could think was, "How the hell do you know that?" He could tell a lot about me just by doing muscle testing. As part of that treatment, he explained to me that my asthma was because my biological father died when I was at the age of one and I did not, at that age, have the capacity to grieve.

Did this healer know your father died or did he sense this during the muscle testing?

My body kind of talked to him through muscle testing. It was fascinating. He did not know that my father died specifically. He was able to go through different ages via muscle testing, and was able to tell me what had happened around those ages. He explained to me that we lock our emotions up in a cage, and if we are able to release those emotions from the cage, then we can heal.

I had known my whole life I had emotional issues with my father dying. I could have talked about it forever and it would not have had the impact on me that this did. I went home and cried for three hours, and I have not had an asthma attack since.

What did he actually do to you during this treatment?

A series of muscle tests to figure out what was going on with different organs, and then, through a series of movements, energy exchanges and questions/answers, he was able to release that emotion caged up in me. It was a really simple technique. I also used this treatment to cure interstitial cystitis. I had a very serious bout of depression that I used this technique to heal from as well.

Was your asthma cured in one treatment?

Yes, he did it in one treatment.

How long was the treatment?

It was about an hour and a half. I don't remember exactly.

Was your asthma triggered by anything other than stress?

The attacks were triggered by stress. As a child I was allergic to dust. Beaches have always been hard for me to visit because the dampness makes it hard to breathe. My husband's family had a family reunion in the desert every year and it was miserable for me.

How severe would you say your asthma was?

I think it ranged from coughing up a lung to not being able to get out of bed for three days.

Do you have any advice for others who are looking for a cure for asthma?

Obviously I am a fan of the holistic methods. There are a lot of holistic methods out there, and it is a matter of finding the one that works for you. I have had several illnesses throughout my life, and in the end, they all can be related to stress. If the full holistic thing is too wacky, do some yoga, do something that calms your stress. Maybe just knowing that the lung is the physical area of depression can help you think through what is making you sad. You may be able to have a conversation with yourself and decide what you need to change.

That is how I approach life. I don't believe that if something comes to me that it is the way it has to be. I believe I can change it. I believe that illness is God's way of saying to me, "Wake up and see that you have to change something." I think if we start to look at what is going on in our lives — are we not eating right, are there people around us who are not healthy for us to be around — we can find answers. Find something that works for you. Healing work was very helpful to me. You have to find that peace. You have to find what on the emotional level is causing that pain.

What did this cost?

He charged by the release. It was not a set cost. He never charged for the first visit, but when you came back for the follow up, you paid him. I think I eventually paid him $100 for that visit. If it didn't work, you didn't pay him, but it always worked. He had a funny way of pricing. He is not doing it anymore — he has passed away.

Do you have any ideas on the type of person this would work for?

I think this is for the person who does not want to be sick anymore. I do not want to be mean, but I do believe there are people who like being sick. They do not want to be well. It gives them the excuse to not do things. It gives them a crutch to lean on. Healing work is definitely not for that person. It is for someone who is willing to look inside themselves. If you are going to go in resistant to change, you are not going to get anything out of it. If you are not willing to change, nothing is going to change. People have to be open to the fact that our bodies are often smarter than doctors; you just have to learn to listen to them.

Anything else you would like to add?

I do not discount the medical side of illness, but I think we also have to look at the emotional side of it. I believe there is a link between depression and the lungs. If you can find a cure for the emotions, very often you can also find a cure for the body.

...

More about Jeanette: www.thecolorwhisperer.com.

#3 Worked with Unresolved Grief, Cured Her Asthma

Edie Weinstein was diagnosed with asthma at the age of four. Through the years, as she relied on the typical Western approach to her illness, she began to learn about the physiological and psychological aspects of the condition. As she improved both her physical health and issues around unresolved grief, Edie was able to cure her asthma. She has not user her inhalers or any asthma medication in over five years.

Here is a bit of her story.

How long did you have asthma before you were completely cured?

I lived with the symptoms of asthma for most of my life, and the symptoms dissipated completely in the last year. The last time I used my inhaler was more than five years ago. I attribute part of my healing to losing weight. I was a lifelong athlete, but in 1992, I had a lot of major life changes. My husband was diagnosed with Hepatitis C, I had an ectopic pregnancy, we lost a home to Hurricane Andrew, and I started putting weight on. It was a gradual process, and I think emotional eating played a role. I sense that the weight put even more of a strain on my lungs and my ability to breathe comfortably. When I lost weight, did more cardio and changed my attitude, that all helped my asthma, along with a lot of other factors.

In the email you sent me, you said that part of your asthma was attributed to unresolved grief. Could you explain a bit about what you meant?

I remember reading about unresolved grief and people telling me over the years that there was a connection between the two. When my grandmother died soon after my fourth birthday, it was like losing a third parent. It is no surprise, when I look back on it through a therapeutic perspective (I have been a therapist for years), that this is when the asthma symptoms started. I have no conscious memory of my parents grieving, although I am sure they did. I know my mom missed her mother her whole life, but she just kept on keeping on. And in the midst of all of this, I started having my first asthma symptoms. On an unconscious level, perhaps I thought, "If my mom does not have to grieve, then neither do I."

My M.O. had always been to run 100 miles per hour, figuratively speaking. When we are doing that, we are not taking in air comfortably, and if I am not fully breathing, then I am not fully living. So that had a lot to do with my asthma also.

What were the first steps you took in curing yourself of asthma?

When I was first diagnosed, I had allergy tests and I was put on steroids. I put on weight as a child from those steroids. When you look at pictures of me from the ages of four to seven, it is evident that I gained weight. As soon as they took me off steroids, I lost the weight. My family doctor was pretty holistic for his time. What he said was that treating asthma was not just about medication, but that exercise and swimming were also excellent ways to help it, so I joined a swim team when I was 11. I did it until I was 18 and then coached for three more years. I think being in the steamy pool environment helped my asthma as well.

In this whole journey were you thinking you were going to completely cure yourself?

No, I just wanted to feel better. I wanted relief and to simply breathe more comfortably. There were times when I felt as if I were suffocating — pretty frightening. Anything that could help with that was beneficial. When I was in college, I started studying mind-body medicine and the ways in which our thoughts contribute to our physiology, as well as the ways in which we see health. I became a vegetarian back then. I don't eat red meat now, but I am not a strict vegetarian, either.

I also started thinking about how the food I ate contributed to my asthma and how I am able to breathe. Also, over the last few years I started to realize that the inhalers were not working.

The other part of curing my asthma was learning to slow down. Meditation helped, yoga helped, focusing on mindfulness helped and noticing my breathing helped. Curing asthma calls for a multi-modal approach.

Is there any one thing that you feel attributed to curing your asthma more than anything else?

I just keep getting back to the mindfulness and the awareness factors. When I am not consciously aware of what I am doing, I speak really quickly, I breathe rapidly and my lungs do not expand and contract fully. To me, asthma is not just physiological, but psychological as well.

How did you cure asthma through healing unprocessed grief?

I do not know if grief is ever completely resolved. I am also a bereavement therapist and a licensed social worker. I have done counseling for others for years around grief. I allow myself to cry when I need to. I allow myself to mourn when I need to. I have had a

23

lot of family members die. My husband died when I was 40. Both of my parents have passed away in the past few years. With every cumulative loss, believe it or not, I have felt like my breathing was better.

I feel like it was hardest initially with my husband, because he was in a coma and on life support for five and a half weeks before he died while awaiting a liver transplant. The asthma was very active then.

When I have been around people with breathing problems, I sometimes empathically take on their symptoms. I know that sounds like cosmic foo-foo, but it is part of my recovery to refrain from taking on someone else's grief. Grief comes up when it does. If I need to cry, I cry. I go to the gym to work out a lot of emotional stuff including grief. If you are at the gym, no one can tell if you are crying or sweating, so it is great. [Laughing] When I practice yoga, sometimes I cry. People cry on the mat a lot. Yoga brings up emotions.

Do you believe that diet overall helped your asthma?

I have a doctor friend who told me that for whatever reason, eating red fruits can contribute to breathing problems, so I stopped eating red apples, raspberries and strawberries, but since then I have gone back to eating them and they do not seem to bother me. But I think the biggest things that contributed to easier breathing for me were to slow down my pace, practice mindfulness, do cardio and lose weight. Because I was not hauling around so much body mass, it helped my breathing.

When you say slowing down and mindfulness, do you consider those two different things?

There is physically slowing down my pace and then there is the mindfulness, the awareness of what I am doing. If you are speaking

100 miles per hour and you cannot catch your breath, you are probably not going to feel your best. When you are rushing through your life, when you are rushing through talking to people and you cannot catch your breath physically and mentally, you can't slow your breathing. I want to be mindful and aware of what I am feeling and what I am doing.

How many years total did you have asthma?

I am 53 now. I have not used my inhaler since my late 40s. I stopped using the inhalers because they were not working. I have not had an asthma attack in I can't tell you how long. I had asthma attacks throughout my whole life where I had to go ER. I have not had bronchitis in years either. In 2005, I believe, was the last time I had serious respiratory issues of any type.

What about advice do you have for others who want to start their journey to curing asthma?

I would say listen to your body, listen to what is it telling you. What are the messages it is giving you? Our bodies are repositories for our emotions. Is your body telling you to take better care of it? Is it telling you to stop smoking? To lose weight? To be away from toxins? To exercise? If you are not able to do rigorous exercise, stretch, swim, walk or float. Do something.

All emotions are "e-motions" — energy in motion. When we are in some kind of motion, we are moving the energy. Be around supportive people who encourage you to take care of yourself and support your lifestyle changes. Be self-compassionate. That is a big one for me. I forget to be compassionate to myself. My inner critic yells at me all day long. I was dancing as fast as I could, which was my M.O. for awhile.

How would someone know if his or her asthma was emotionally exacerbated or induced?

I think it takes a level of conscious awareness to know that. It is a matter of having an awareness of when you are having hard time breathing. People should ask themselves, "When do I notice I have challenges in breathing?" For a lot of people, asthma is exercise-induced. I was the opposite, in that exercise made it better. I noticed that the times when I was most likely to have the symptoms were when I was upset, when I had an argument or when there was a trauma. I noticed that I was inclined to feel like I had a hard time breathing.

Did you use supplements, vitamins, acupuncture — anything like that?

No.

Did you feel anything you tried did not help?

Occasionally, the inhalers would help me catch my breath, but overall they did not make a difference in helping me cure myself. I do not like dissing medical treatments, and I am not telling anyone not to take their medicine or not to go to their doctor. However, I am saying to be aware of how you are feeling and what is and is not working, and then discuss these things with your health-care practitioner.

Does it surprise you that you are cured of asthma?

No, not at all. When I listen to my body and I listen to its instructions, and when I am in connection with my body and having a dialogue with it — it gets better

...

More about Edie: www.liveinjoy.org.

#4 Changed Her Life, Cured Her Asthma

Katrina Love Senn was once 60 pounds overweight. She suffered with asthma, eczema, Chronic Fatigue Syndrome and thyroid issues, among other chronic diseases. When her body collapsed 15 years, ago her doctors wanted to prescribe "experimental prescription medicine." Her intuition guided her to say no to the medication. Acting on this intuition, she refused the doctors' medicine and instead went on her own healing journey. Katrina now lives 100 percent free of asthma and all her previous symptoms.

Here is a bit of her story.

What was the breaking point that made you want to make such significant changes to your health and life?

My asthma originally started when I was six years old with my first asthma attack, the result of a severe allergic reaction to animals. Over the years, I was put on all different types of inhalers and medications. As I got older, the drugs and inhalers got stronger.

From a young age, I suffered with not only asthma, but also allergies, eczema and other health problems. As a child, I was "in and out" of different doctors' offices with my asthma, seeking information to improve my breathing and stop my asthma attacks. I thought my body was my enemy.

This caused me to develop an unhealthy relationship with food. From my early teens, I was always trying to lose weight or go on the next diet, but the problem was I loved food about as much as I hated exercise. I was the sort of person who found it was really easy to gain weight and really hard to lose it. So, in an effort to lose weight, I started dieting.

For me, dieting was always about taking away my favorite foods; it was always about restrictions. Diets worked for a few days until I would get stressed, hungry, emotional or just be like, "Screw it," and tell myself that the diet would begin again on Monday.

My breaking point came just days before my 20th birthday. When I was just 19 years of age, I was at a conference in Australia. On the day I was supposed to speak, I woke up in the morning and I could not even open my eyes or move my body. I had zero energy. The doctors came to see me and immediately put me on the next plane back home, to New Zealand.

It was at this point that I knew that I had to start doing things differently. I realized that I needed to make significant changes to my health and my life. My mind had been running the show up to that point.

When my body collapsed, it served as a very painful wake-up call. At the time, I would have told you it was my breakdown moment, but with the benefit of hindsight, I feel fortunate that it was able to serve as my real "breakthrough" moment.

How did you go from unhealthy habits to learning healthy habits?

My doctors could not figure out what was wrong with me. They wanted to put me on experimental medication. After all these years of struggling with medication for my asthma, I had the feeling that my body was trying to tell me something — it seemed obvious that more drugs were not the answer.

From there, I started asking myself, "If I am not going to take the experimental medicine, then what else could I possibly do?'" I talked to my mom and she was really supportive about helping me to go more of a natural route to heal my body. I started reading about nutrition and the importance of vitamins and minerals for the body and our health, and the role they play in creating energy naturally. These were things I had never even thought about. From there, my research took me to different natural health practitioners, including homeopaths, iridologists and reflexologists, but it was not until I met a naturopath who explained to me that food can be used to help the body and food can be used to harm the body that I saw a much bigger picture. She gave me the hope that I could heal my body from within.

Was food the primary mechanism you used to heal yourself?

Yes. I have come to understand that healing ourselves is possible. I like to break the healing journey into three distinct parts: healing your body, healing your mind and healing your emotions.

Food is certainly a powerful healing tool and it was one that I used to physically heal myself. However, always remember that the conversation around healing is much bigger than just food. But when you are just starting on your healing journey, know that food is a great place to start. It has the ability to make a huge difference to your energy levels, especially when you turn your attention toward eating whole foods. When you do this, you allow healing to happen naturally. I started my healing journey by focusing only on healing my body, but then, a few short years later, I went on to address the mental and emotional aspects of healing, or what I call the "inner world."

I realized that to heal myself 100 percent, I also needed to look within and heal my "inner world" of thoughts and feelings as well. What this meant for me in practice was that for me to really heal, I also needed to give myself permission to let go of my identity of being an asthmatic. With this awareness and shift in consciousness, I realized how much I had been holding myself back from life, because literally (for whatever reason) I couldn't or wouldn't breathe

31

life in. I realized that I had been suppressing my feelings, such as my fear, my frustration and my sadness.

As I became more conscious of how my internal world was affecting my ability to breathe, I started to make different distinctions along the way.

As you are going on this healing journey, are you thinking, "I am going to do this particular thing to cure asthma and this other thing to cure Chronic Fatigue Syndrome and this other thing to lose weight," or was it a one approach healing that in the end healed everything?

At this stage in my journey, I was so sick that I had had to quit university for a few months. My body had completely collapsed, and I was bed-ridden, sleeping for up to 20 hours a day. My mom was spoon-feeding me soup. In those long, uncomfortable weeks, I remember just wanting to get some energy back in my body again.

What I did learn is that as I started to eat the right kind of foods, all my different types of "diseases," or symptoms labeled as disease, were finally able to start healing as well. My naturopath explained to me that my body was particularly sensitive. When you are sensitive, you react easily to stress and stressful environments. In addition, certain kinds of foods stress the physical body. As I started to detoxify my body by eating a mainly whole-foods diet (i.e., no processed foods, dairy, wheat or refined sugars) combined with liver-supporting supplements and adaptogenics, or calming herbs, my energy started to return. I learned what foods were stimulating and aggravating to my body, and I made the transition to eating foods that were nourishing and healing for my body. Now I can eat anything in moderation. But I first had to allow my body time to heal. This allowed my body to come back into balance naturally.

When you (or your body) are stressed, you go into the "fight or flight" state and everything becomes more alert, much more heightened. The body is always, always trying to talk to us, and we need to learn to listen to it if we are to stay healthy.

Do you believe the diet you were on would help anyone with asthma?

Everyone is unique, but if you have asthma or any health problem it is important to know that food is either healing or hurting your body. Certain foods heal whilst certain foods harm your body. You need to find out which foods do what for your body. The thing that is so wonderful about our world today is that so much information is at the tip of our fingers. But even with so much information available on the topic of healing, for many people, knowing "what to eat" can be one of the most challenging things to figure out. We all have different ideas around it — around what is healthy and what is not. What you should eat and what you should not. It is important to break through the dogma and also question the advertising and marketing claims you hear or see. If you are not sure what to believe, a good trick is to "follow the money." By that, I mean find out who is telling you that you should eat a certain type of food. If they are likely to financially gain from your buying and eating that product, then research it more. Find healthy food brands that you can trust, read labels and make sure you can pronounce all the words on the label. Chances are that if you can't, you probably don't want to eat it.

One of the things that I learned when I first started learning about food was about the nightshade family – eggplants, peppers, tomatoes, potatoes — any of these foods really increased my sensitivity to asthma, and it was only through experimenting and seeing what would happen by not eating them and seeing what would happen when I did eat them that I was able to see how these different foods were affecting me.

When you take a healing approach, you are taking the time to learn about yourself and to educate yourself about what is right for you. This is about taking responsibility for your health as well as your life. We live in a quick-fix world, and it is easy to want to look for the quick fix. What I have found is that in the long-term, it is much more effective to take a sustainable approach to your health. Just take baby steps, and over time, the unhealthy patterns replace the healthy ones. If you build a house on a solid foundation, it will stand strong for years.

When you are on a healing journey, there will come a point where you will never need to worry about asthma or any kind of chronic disease ever again. Even if I had the symptoms now, I could look within and think, "What healing tools do I need to draw upon to bring myself back into balance?"

On your website you mention dehydration played a role in your asthma.

I think many people think if you drink a lot of water it will solve a lot of problems, but when the body is toxic — and we live in a world with high toxicity — we may not even be able to absorb the water. You need to detoxify the body by eating whole foods and maybe doing a cleanse, so that the body can start to absorb water easily and naturally. When I was living on coffee and processed foods, I could not hear my body's cry or request for water. As I started to eat more fruits, vegetables, nuts, seeds and whole foods, I became much more conscious of when my body was thirsty and how much water I needed to drink.

To be honest, in the beginning of my journey, I did not really like drinking plain water. My body was very used to sugar. So, one thing I would do is add things into my glass of water to try and give it some interesting tastes and flavors. I added in extras such as cucumber, mint, pineapple pieces or freshly squeezed lemon juice.

Spicing up water to make it more interesting definitely helped me drink it more. I had a two-liter bottle filled with water on my desk, which also made it easy to remember to drink lots of water throughout the day.

How did you know there was a connection between dehydration and your asthma?

To be honest, I can't remember. I think as I started to educate myself about food, I realized that my body needed water to cleanse and purify itself. Asthma or any chronic disease is a buildup of internal toxicity that is foreign to the body. Drinking water can help your body to detoxify naturally, so as the body begins to detoxify naturally, all the symptoms of asthma such as the wheeziness, the excess phlegm and mucous, the gasping for air and the difficulty in breathing can release as well.

How much water were you drinking?

Before I went on my healing journey, I was not drinking a lot of water — maybe just a couple of glasses a day. But the funny thing was that I don't remember feeling particularly thirsty. This is probably because when anyone is living on a highly processed diet, as I was, and is having a lot of stimulants throughout the day, the body is not able to register thirst very well. In those days, my body was mainly fueled by coffee and sugar. There are a lot of great books on the power of water to help aid the healing process. I urge people who are suffering with any form of chronic disease to include water as a part of their healing journey.

How long did it take until you did not need to use your inhaler?

My health crisis happened in 1997, and it took a couple of years of healing to stop using my inhaler, to completely heal my asthma and lose 60 pounds at the same time. The last time I used my inhaler was around 1999 or 2000.

I remember a great moment at the end of 2002: I went on an Outward Bound outdoor leadership course. I had to have a doctor's certification to do it. I had not been to a doctor in years. During my visit, the doctor had me blow into a peak flow meter to measure the speed of air I could exhale from my lungs. He took other tests, and at the end of my visit said to me, "I am happy to tell you, you are 100 percent free of asthma."

Did exercise help with your asthma?

To be honest, I don't really think it played a big part. I didn't like running when I was younger, and I don't like it today. I like walking or hiking. It is important to move your body gently, but break free of the mindset of "burning calories" or "you have to do cardio" to get results. In fact, cardio stresses out your adrenal glands, which when functioning normally, produce a number of hormones that support our growth, ability to handle stress and kidney functions. So if you are already feeling emotionally stressed or exhausted, doing stressful exercise could compound the strain on your body.

Be gentle with yourself and move your body gently. Stretch and breathe. Then smile. Have fun and do things that you love. Remember that life is short. Go after your dreams.

What advice do you have for someone who is looking to cure or heal asthma?

There are so many things that you can start to do today to feel better and heal your asthma.

One, eat a healing diet that is right for your body. In my book, Losing Weight Is a Healing Journey, I speak about stimulants such as fast food, coffee and sugar as being artificial energy sources. They fill you up, they look like food but yet your body doesn't recognize them as food.

Two, detoxify your body so that you can eliminate foods that are aggravating your body and replace them with foods that can heal you and your body. Eating in this way is easy. For me, it is all about food freedom. I call this "substitution not deprivation." If you want to eat ice cream, find a non-dairy ice cream. Instead of processed cow's milk, substitute it for organic non-dairy milk instead. Also, experiment with replacing any vegetables in the nightshade family [with those that are not]

Three, have as much of a clean green diet as you can and by that I mean eating lots of green real, whole foods that are easy on the digestion.Green foods from vegetables & super foods such as chlorella, spirulina, barley grass and wheatgrass. I include green foods in my salads, soups, smoothies and stews. I always encourage people to aim for 50 percent green foods on their plate each meal.

Four, hydrate as much as you can. When you are properly hydrated, the body is not going to be craving the stimulants and the refined processed foods.

Five, understand that food cravings equal nutritional hunger. We have not talked about supplements, but it is good to find really good supplements. I found I was really deficient in vitamins B and C, as well as magnesium. When you are on a junk-food diet, you are really going to be depleted. When you drink a lot of alcohol, your liver can be weakened as well. You want to deal with the root cause of the symptoms you are having.

In the medical world, we are used to putting a Band-Aid over the problem to mask the symptoms. By contrast, with the healing approach, we look at what is causing the symptoms and how can we go about healing the root cause of the problem. True healing can only happen from within when you begin to detoxify your body and start eating, drinking, thinking and doing things that are nourishing for you and your life.

Could you talk about how you changed your mindset and identity in association with asthma?

In a funny kind of way, having asthma served me. What I mean by that is that quite often, my asthma gave me the excuses I needed to get out of doing the things I didn't want to do. I used "having asthma" as a reason to get out of P.E. classes at school and to not to have to participate in swimming classes, sports days, running competitions and other school sporting events. I came to rely on my asthma as a crutch.

It was only when I started to heal my body that I realized a lot of those crutches were not necessary any longer. They had helped me when I was younger, but then I realized I didn't need them anymore. As I started to heal, I gave myself the opportunity to learn how to have the confidence to communicate my needs, whereas before I would not have the confidence to express myself or allow myself to be heard. In many ways, for whatever reason, I did not feel safe to be me. But as I got more confident and got to connect with other like-minded people, I realized it was OK to be me.

As this happened, my world started to expand and I found within me the confidence I had been looking for all along. This allowed me to start connecting with my spiritual, creative and artistic self. What I have realized is that my sensitivity is my gift. Today it is my sensitivity that enables me to do work that I love. Without it, I wouldn't be able to teach, heal, write or speak in the way that I do.

After you have changed your diet to a supportive and healing one, you can work on identifying and releasing the mental/emotional aspects of being an asthmatic. I remember — even after I had not had asthma for many months — the fear and panic at the thought of going away without taking my inhaler, and still looking for the courage to leave home without it.

Do you have any ideas on the root cause of your asthma?

No, I really have no idea. It may have been about being different in my family. Or it may have been about being noticed in my family, because my asthma did bring me a lot of attention (not consciously of course). A part of the healing process was about learning how to get attention in positive ways and realizing I did not "need my asthma" to get attention, as I was able to attract it in more empowering ways.

Anything else you would like to add?

If you have asthma today, just know that it is totally possible to heal it. The guru lives within. It is great to hear other people's stories of success. Fill your mind with them. Have fun in your life and do whatever it takes to get yourself connected and inspired to follow your dreams. Come on a yoga retreat with me!

Just remember that whatever you want to do, you can do it. No matter what and no matter how many specialists and doctors tell you otherwise. Just know that you can do it. If you keep looking, you will find the answers. Life is a journey; when you realize that, all the things we struggle with are only here to help us to break through to deeper levels of understanding. On the other side is freedom, and it's an amazing feeling. You deserve that feeling.

…

More about Katrina: www.katrinalovesenn.com.

#5 Doctor Who Cures Asthma with Rib Alignments and More

Dr. Dale Peterson spent his first 20 years as an M.D. practicing as most doctors in the United States do: diagnosing "what" patients had, and then prescribing medication. Then he realized the key to actually curing patients was in not only understanding "what" patients had but "why" they had it. Since then, Dr. Peterson has helped many patients overcome and cure numerous diseases, including asthma in adults and children.

Here is a bit of his story.

How do you define asthma?

It is generally defined as a reversible spasm in the bronchial tubes. The general symptoms are wheezing, shortness of breath and sometimes a dry cough.

What do you mean by a "reversible spasm?"

I mean that the spasm in the bronchial tubes comes and goes. A person can have a spasm in the bronchial tubes where the muscles have tightened and the air is not moving well, but we can reverse it with medication — or sometimes it reverses itself — but by reversible, we mean that the bronchial tubes do not stay in constant spasm.

What are the different ways you as an M.D. can help patients prevent that bronchial spasm?

There are a number of things that can happen. Most individuals are only aware of certain medications, called bronchodilators, which contain adrenaline-like substances, but there are a number of nutritional things I help people work with that are very helpful. Magnesium is the body's natural muscle relaxant. When people supplement magnesium on a regular basis, they have far fewer asthma attacks as a result of those muscles in the bronchial tube being more relaxed and therefore less likely to go into spasm.

I will also have someone use an adrenal-support formula.

The adrenal glands are the stress glands of the body. It seems that modern living is filled with stress. There are nutrients that are available that support the adrenal glands. Supporting the ability of the adrenals to produce hormones can decrease the frequency of attacks.

Asthma is an inflammatory disease. If you can control the inflammation, you can markedly decrease the severity and frequency of asthma attacks. The omega-3 oils commonly found in fish and other sources can decrease the severity and frequency of asthma attacks. We know that people who have a tendency to have asthma also have lower levels of vitamin C, so we use a lot of antioxidant supplements as well. There are a lot of different things people can do to decrease the severity and frequency of asthma attacks before I resort to the medications. A lot of people come off the medications when they start giving their bodies that support.

What are the things that cause inflammation?

One of the main things is the standard American diet, which seems to be high in animal products and processed foods. This diet tends to lead to deficiency in omega-3s and therefore produces inflammation. Lack of sleep can lead to inflammation. Irritants from the air — cigarette smoke, for example — can lead to inflammation, asthma and asthma attacks.

There was a unique situation in my practice that led me to a unique cure for asthma. I am particularly sensitive when seeing an adult who comes in with symptoms of asthma who has not had these asthma symptoms in the past. I had a patient come in who was wheezing and had shortness of breath and difficulty with exertion. He had a rib out of place. A rib not moving freely can trigger a bronchial spasm as well. If a misplaced rib is able to move freely, the wheezing goes away, and that person is not condemned to lifetime use of inhalers and other medications.

How would someone know if their rib was misaligned and causing this asthmatic response?

Via examination. I have people lie down on their stomach, and I check to see if their heels align when they are lying flat. If the ribs are out of place, it will make it appear as if one leg is longer than the other, which it really is not — it is just pulled up because of the tightness on that side of the spine. I ask the patient to take breaths in and out. If the heels move as they breathe instead of remaining stationary, it tells me that something is hung up, which is preventing them from moving freely. Unfortunately, I was never taught this in medical school. I learned it from a friendly neighborhood chiropractor who taught me.

What causes a rib misalignment?

Several things can, such as falling, bumping one's side, lifting a weight or twisting to one side. It can cause a rib to be hung up, locked up and not move freely.

Is the only way to fix a misaligned rib with a chiropractic procedure or could this be fixed via exercise or other methods?

While it's possible that a misaligned rib might slip back into place spontaneously, I always fix it when someone presents with the challenge. I don't know of any particular exercise or home maneuver that will consistently resolve the issue.

Is there a way to reverse asthma permanently?

That is a tricky question, because there are individuals who have a pre-disposition to bronchospasm or wheezing, which we call asthma. If they are paying attention to their diet, if they are using the supplements, often I do not see them back in my office. It does not mean the pre-disposition is gone. It means they are no longer bothered by the pre-disposition to the spasm in the bronchial tubes.

If someone was looking for a doctor like you, what sort of qualifications, approaches and methods should they be looking for?

It might be helpful if you understand how I approach disease. In medical school, I was taught to diagnose a person by finding out what they have. Mid-career, I changed. If you would have come to me in the first half of my career and given me a list of symptoms you were having, I would have looked you over and I would have been trying to answer, "What do you have?" I could put a name on it. That would be my diagnosis. But asking, "What do you have?" is the wrong question. Now, in my practice, it is not about "what" but about "why."

The physician should be able to give a reasonable answer when asked the question, "Why do I have this condition?" He or she should also be able to recommend measures that will address and potentially correct the cause of the health challenge you are facing, rather than simply prescribing a drug to relieve the symptoms you are experiencing.

Symptoms are like the warning lights on a car dashboard. If a red light that says "oil" appears, it can be put out by clipping the wire leading to it. Unfortunately, serious engine damage may result if the reason the light appeared isn't addressed. Taking a drug to relieve a symptom without identifying the cause is like clipping the wire to the warning light. A much more serious condition may appear in the future.

Do you believe your approach is the standard approach in Western medicine?

Absolutely not. My approach is what I call a mechanism approach in which I ask, "What is the mechanism that is causing this, and how do we approach that?" Western medicine takes a symptomatic approach, where you say you are wheezing and they give you a bronchodilator, but it is not about figuring out what is causing the problem and then addressing that.

What do you think are the side effects of the long-term use of the inhalers?

It is not so much that I am concerned about the negative impact of the drugs, but about the long-term effects of the inflammation. If the lining of the bronchial tubes is swollen and inflamed, it will cause breakdown over time. My mother, who was 85, passed away a few weeks ago. The cause of death was her lifelong asthma. She developed it early in life. Over time, her bronchial tubes broke down, and her asthma turned into emphysema. Had she known earlier on in her life about various ways to reduce inflammation, she may have been spared getting on oxygen and ultimately dying in the process.

I am very sorry to hear about your mom.

She was ready to go. As death goes, hers was the most ideal I can imagine. The big thing is when we start addressing the underlying causes of an illness, then we can really address things that will add to the quality and quantity of a person's life.

I am interested in the reaction from your counterparts in the Western medical world regarding your approach.

They think I am weird. Obviously, individual thinking is not tolerated very well in American medicine. It has degenerated into a cookbook approach. When someone comes in with lupus, for example, it is a cookbook approach — "If you have lupus, these are the medicines we prescribe" — rather than asking why they might have it. Have they developed a chronic infection? Do they have a reaction to food? What can we address that might have the answer? American medicine is not open to addressing nutritional concerns or structural concerns. In American medicine, doctors like me are tolerated, but not accepted or endorsed.

The best example I can give you is that I have been in medicine for 40 years. I graduated from medical school in 1972. In the mid-90s, I gradually started taking this mechanism approach and truly saw people starting to get well, as opposed to degenerating over time. When I finally started seeing people get well, I had been a medical professor at the University of Oklahoma and taught for many years. When I started teaching this approach, the university stopped sending me students. After I stopped seeing students for five years, even though I requested them, they pulled my professorship, saying I was inactive and no longer had the title. It was that sort of, "You are not part of the club anymore. You are not following the recipe of diagnose–prescribe, diagnose-prescribe."

I have heard asthma has to do with a weakened immune and/or digestive system. Do you have any thoughts on that?

There is an autoimmune component to asthma in which the body is reacting to certain substances, but ultimately, in most cases, the inflammation is the real key. If we can find the cause of that and deal with it, then we will likely see some results.

You talked about magnesium as being a good supplement for inflammation. What are some naturally occurring sources where magnesium is available?

The problem is that there are not a lot of naturally occurring sources of magnesium in our food. People are going to get it primarily from whole grains, but that is not a natural part of the American diet. To really get the magnesium that a body needs, you are going to have to supplement it, and usually with 400 to 600 milligrams of magnesium citrate or magnesium aspartate. Those are both forms of magnesium that are well-absorbed and used by the body.

What advice do you have for adults who have had lifelong, chronic asthma?

The big message is that it is not too late. We can really see significant improvement anytime someone makes positive changes. If someone is 43 and has history of asthma and they are on an assortment of medications, we can talk to them about diet, we can talk to them about drinking purified water as their primary drink and we can talk about keeping them hydrated, which will seriously decrease inflammation. Mild dehydration is very common in the United States. We push drinking more water. We are cleaning up their diet. We give supplements. I have seen many adults not only decrease their amount of medication, but get off of it entirely and live symptom-free. Does that mean it is cured? It is cured in the sense that what was present is no longer there. If they stop doing what they did to bring resolution to the problem, the symptoms will appear.

Is your approach different when treating children with asthma?

No, not really.

What about exercise? Are there any exercises you do or do not recommend for people with asthma?

People who have asthma can be very successful athletes. We have had a number of Olympic gold-medal athletes who have been asthmatic. What I tell asthmatics is that the exercises they do will be easier if they are in the horizontal position. Many of the Olympic athletes have been bikers and swimmers. It is much easier on the body if you are in the horizontal position. You do not get as much spasm in the airways for whatever reason when the body is in that position. People will have more problems in basketball and soccer — where they are continually running — as opposed to start-and-stop sports like baseball and tennis. If you are going to be in competitive sports, look for where your body can be horizontal. You will have a lot more success.

That is interesting, because a lot of asthmatics have problems when they lay down to go to sleep at night.

Yes, it is interesting. When one lies down in bed at night, it tends to increase the spasm in the airways. There is something about leaning forward. It might just be the difference between being on your back and being on your stomach.

Do you ever recommend specific breathing exercises for asthma?

Chances are that unless someone has played a wind instrument, they have never been taught to breathe properly. Most people I see, and asthmatics are no exception, tend to breathe from the top of their chest, and that is not effective breathing. You are supposed to breathe from your abdomen. If you are breathing properly, your stomach will move out as you breathe in and move in when you breathe out. If you do this, your breathing will be much more efficient and that will be much more beneficial. You can actually strengthen the diaphragm with these exercises by putting weights on your stomach and moving them up and down while you breathe in and out.

Is there anything else you would like to add?

One thing that I find very useful is systemic enzymes. They are very useful in reducing inflammation in the body. When people are struggling with frequent asthma attacks, I often have them use systemic enzymes. It takes quite a few. I use PanZymes or Wobenzym. There is another one called Vitalzym. I have them use four to six capsules, three times a day, but it really starts reducing the inflammation, which can be the difference between struggling with asthma attacks and leading a relatively normal life.

…

More about Dr. Peterson: www.drdalepeterson.com/index.php.

#6 From Near-Fatal Asthma Attack to Inhaler-Free for 17 Years

Jim Quinlan was diagnosed with asthma when he was in his 30s. Initially, he was reluctant to use the prescribed inhaler. With time, he was terrified to leave home without it. Jim's asthma became so severe that an asthma attack almost killed him. Through his own research and perseverance, Jim determined that his severe asthma was caused by a bacterial infection. With this knowledge Jim started taking antibiotics and cured himself in 1995. He has not used his inhaler or any asthma medication since.

Here is a bit of his story.

How was having a near fatal asthma attack a turning point in your life?

After I got out of the hospital we decided it was time to do something radical so we sold our house [in Michigan] and moved to Florida to try a different climate. Unfortunately the Florida climate didn't make any difference. Right after the move is when our pharmacist friend found Dr. Hahn's research and forwarded it to us.

What was your reaction to being diagnosed as an adult with asthma?

Initially, I was quite angry with the doctor. I just thought, "There is no way I have asthma. This guy does not know what he is talking about." He gave me an albuterol inhaler. I tried it and I hated it, but eventually, I started using it. I got to the point where I was terrified to leave home without it.

At what point did you think your asthma problems were being caused by bacteria?

After my near-fatal asthma attack in 1995, a friend of mine who was a pharmacist saw an interesting medical-journal article written by Dr. David Hahn. He has done extensive research on asthma and bacteria.

How was it determined that you had a Chlamydia pneumoniae bacteria infection?

At the time, there were some crude tests that just indicated that your body was at one time exposed to the [Chlamydia pneumoniae] bacteria. That was how Dr. Hahn determined that the treatment could be helpful. Currently, doctors no longer do testing because the available tests are just not accurate enough.

What were the antibiotics you took? At what dosage did you take them, and how long did it take to become cured?

I took Zithromax (azithromycin) at 1,000 milligrams per week for 14 weeks. However, there's evidence that it takes a lot longer than 14 weeks to work for most people. Several doctors are prescribing Zithromax for up to a year and using a variety of dosing. It takes a lot to completely eradicate your body of these bacteria. Having a strong immune system also helps.

Were there any significant side effects with taking antibiotics for a long period of time? Did you find that to be the case?

Not at all. I was not taking a lot of antibiotics. The dose I took is the standard dose that they give to people with acne. I have heard of people having occasional mild stomach problems with the antibiotics, but nothing severe. There is another doctor, Dr. Fred Wagschul, and he prescribes antibiotics for a year for treating asthma. He believes that taking antibiotics for this long is not a problem.

Were you taking probiotics at the same time that you were taking antibiotics?

A lot of people do, but I did not.

Did you try any other approaches to help or cure your asthma?

There was nothing that I saw that would work for me. There are different types of asthma. I had severe and relentless asthma. I was constantly wheezing. I was taking a lot of medications just to try to breathe. I tried to eat healthier and do more exercise. One thing I did do was a partial anti-candida diet, which may have helped. It involves removing excessive sugar from your diet to keep excessive yeast out of your body, which can cause flare-ups. There was a good book I read — the name was The Yeast Connection.

On your website, you indicate that Dr. Hahn is now not recommending taking a blood test to detect Chlamydia pneumoniae, as the test can be inaccurate. Do you know the best way to determine if you have a Chlamydia pneumonia infection?

If you have severe asthma and conventional treatment is not working, then it is recommended you go for the antibiotic treatment, because you have nothing to lose. It makes sense. It is a safe approach. Usually, you can tell pretty quickly if you are going to be a good candidate for the antibiotics because you start to feel better in a short period of time. I have people write to me and say that within just a couple weeks of taking the antibiotics, they can breathe normally again. The problem with this is the bacteria does come back until you completely eradicate it from your system.

Do you have any thoughts on the average time it takes to eradicate Chlamydia pneumonia from your system?

I don't know. I hear from people, but I do not hear all the stories. I kind of agree with Dr. Wagschul regarding taking the antibiotics for a year. Dr. Hahn does it for 14 weeks at a time, multiple times. Dr. Wagschul recommends a year with one or two different kinds of antibiotics. Dr. Wagschul claims a 95 to 99 percent success rate. I think closer to a year is important once you realize how serious this bacteria is and how hard it is to eradicate.

As I read new research from Dr. Wilmore Webley and others, I have learned how this bacteria can replicate in your body and protect itself from antibiotics, which is why you may need to use several different kinds of antibiotics to eradicate it from your system. They are finding that this bacteria can also cause heart disease, A.L.S., M.S., rheumatoid arthritis and Alzheimer's. They have found these bacteria in parts of the brain where Alzheimer's is. It is hard to prove. The studies are just beginning.

Do you know if there is a time lapse in between the 14-week treatments? Do you know approximately how many 14-week treatments people typically take?

Everybody is different. A lot depends on how strong your immune system is. Some can get better after 14 weeks, but from what I hear, at least a couple rounds is more normal. As far as the time lapse is concerned, after I took my 14 weeks, I felt the bacteria was still somewhat with me. My immune system was strengthened by the antibiotics, so it took several more months until I realized my asthma was completely gone.

What are the signs people should look for in determining if there is a high chance that they have a Chlamydia pneumonia infection?

If you have adult onset of asthma and/or if all of the sudden you have really bad asthma, there is a very high probability you may have it. If you have had mild asthma all your life, then it's hard to tell if this treatment would apply to you or not — but it might.

Does Chlamydia pneumonia-induced asthma produce constant asthmatic symptoms, or does it come and go with days, weeks or seasons?

It is severe. You are always on edge, not knowing where your next breath is coming from. It was always, for me, really difficult to breathe at night. But everyone has different triggers that set it off.

After the antibiotic treatment is complete, is there a way to test to see if you have eradicated Chlamydia pneumonia from your system?

The symptoms are gone. That is the true test. There are a lot of researchers around the world that are working on this, and they may have come up with something by now. I am not an expert on this. These microbiologists are the ones to answer those questions.

On your website, you discuss how many doctors are reluctant about this treatment. Do you have any suggestions on how people could have a conversation with their doctor about getting antibiotics to treat their asthma?

Back in the day, doctors were a lot more close-minded. I am hearing nowadays that there is so much research out there about this that doctors are becoming more aware of it as a viable way to treat asthma. A lot of people are bringing in the research and showing their doctors. Seventeen years ago, it was really difficult to find an open-minded doctor.

It was 17 years ago that you stopped using an inhaler?

Yes.

Do you carry one with you now?

Never. For the first six months after, I always had one around me because I thought, "This can't be."

Do you have any idea where you picked up this bacteria?

It started out as a really bad cold. I was at a restaurant one night, and I remember being in the lobby and all of these people were coughing and sick and the next day I got really sick. It was one of those really bad colds that gets in your lungs and won't go away. After a few months of it not going away, I went to the doctor, was diagnosed with asthma and got an inhaler.

What advice do you have for people who have just been diagnosed with asthma? Do you recommend they immediately look at this antibiotic solution?

I can't recommend anything because I am not a doctor, and I am really careful about that. The only thing I can say is having severe asthma is pure hell. The quality of life goes right down the tubes because you can't do anything without fear of a massive asthma attack and not being able to breathe. I would probably try conventional medicine first, and if it doesn't work — or if it keeps getting worse — I would consider Dr. Hahn's antibiotic treatment.

Can you begin to describe how the quality of your life has changed since being cured of asthma?

I can do whatever I want. I hiked the Appalachian Trail. I hiked the Florida Everglades. It is fun to be able to push yourself physically and mentally and not have to worry about having to breathe. I'm also entered in the next WaterTribe Everglades Challenge, which is a 300-mile small-boat race from St. Petersburg, Florida, cutting through the Everglades to Key Largo. I'll be in a small Hobie kayak with a sail.

Is there anything else you would like to add?

The important thing to understand is why it takes longer for the antibiotics to help some people. I would recommend looking at the research about bio-films and how this bacteria can protect itself in your body. I think a lot of us have Chlamydia pneumonia in us, but our immune system is strong and can protect us from it. Other people do not have the same defenses. In the future, I think we are going to hear that this is the cause of many chronic diseases. Also, this treatment has been successfully used to cure children with severe asthma as well as adults.

An excellent book by Dr. David Hahn on this subject will be published in September or October of 2012. I highly recommend anyone interested in this research to read this informative book. I will post the link on my website as soon as it's available.

…

More about Jim: www.asthmastory.com.

#7 Cured Asthma with Energy Work

Sheila was diagnosed with asthma around the age of 12. After living with asthma for decades, she learned of a man by the name of Tom Tam who was healing people of some of life's most serious diseases. She decided to see how he could help her asthma. A few months after attending his classes, her Western medical doctor took her off her asthma medication, and she has not needed it since.

Here is a bit of her story.

Tell me about the journey to meeting Tom Tam.

I was diagnosed with asthma when I was a kid. Then I was a teenager who smoked, which did not help. I would have asthma attacks so severe that I would have to go the hospital for a few days and be hooked up to an IV. Interestingly, when I started to smoke, my asthma was not cured, but it was more masked. When I quit smoking 20 years later, my asthma really reared its ugly head. I was taking a steroid inhaler every morning — I really couldn't function without it — and often was prescribed prednisone to get me through a tough asthma attack.

I was introduced to Tom Tam last year. He is an amazing man. I saw him for both his energy-healing class and for acupuncture. He has helped me with my asthma to the point where I do not take any of my asthma medications at all. I don't remember the last time I have been to the hospital. He has been an amazing find for me. He can't cure everybody, but has a great track record. Tom Tam has been a huge help to many people, and he has been a huge help to me.

I would go to him on a Thursday and get acupuncture and attend a healing class. Then I would go to one of his energy-healing classes on Sunday. I had acupuncture once a week. Now I have acupuncture once every five weeks. I spent the first few months going every Sunday to his energy-healing class, and now I have been only going to his energy class every five weeks, or once a month.

If I went to a new doctor, I would say that I have had a history of asthma, but if asked if I was asthmatic, I would say no. Previously, I would have to leave dinner parties because I would have an asthmatic attack. I was that sensitive. I am so grateful to Tom Tam.

Could you explain the energy-healing classes?

The very first class I went to was at the Spaulding Rehabilitation Hospital in Boston. I had no idea what to expect. There were about 100 people in the room. He goes around the room and asks people how they are doing. He knows a lot of these people because he has been working with them for so long. He asks how recent medical tests went. Many of these people have very serious diseases. When he asked me, I told him I had asthma.

Then Tom Tam and about 10 other people are in the front of the room, banging this little acupuncture doll each of them have with a silver hammer. He bangs the doll on the point that corresponds with the one you mentioned as being problematic. For example, let's say a patient had asthma — he would call out the coordinating number for a lung point, and then everyone in the room with a doll will bang on that particular point with their silver hammer.

What he is doing is taking universal energy and directing it to whatever unique problem individuals in the room have. I know that sounds strange, but all I can tell you is it works. You can see people when he is working on them. You can see their faces get red from the energy. I did not feel that, but I definitely felt something. Banging on these dolls is his way of directing whatever you want to say — energy, divine healing — to a certain point, and that is all it is.

How long does he do this for each person?

Not long. Maybe 30 or 45 seconds. For example, the woman in front of me, who was kind of cranky, said she had shoulder surgery and could only lift her arm five inches. So he calls out a coordinating shoulder point and everyone starts banging on this doll in this particular point for about 45 seconds. When he was done he asked her to lift her arm. She could lift her arm 10 inches. She said, "I still cannot lift my arm above my head." And he said, "You can lift it twice as far as you could before."

I was amazed at that, and there were all sorts of stories like that all around the room. He does not charge for these classes. He asks for a donation. People put maybe $10 in a box. It is not about the money to him.

He helped cure a woman who had a vision problem. She was a doctor. She quit everything and went to work for him.

Did you feel anything when he had the class hit a point on the doll for you?

At the first class I went to, I felt something. Since then I have not felt a lot, maybe a little tingle, but I do not feel a lot. But I can take a deep breath now, that is for sure.

After the class, how do you feel an hour or two later?

I don't feel any different, and that is the amazing thing — but the difference is, I don't take any asthma medication or any medication anymore. For the first time in my life, I don't take medication.

Was it immediately after that first class that you stopped taking the medication?

It was a couple of months into going to these energy-healing classes and getting acupuncture that I went to my primary-care doctor, who is an osteopath. I told him that I'd cut down taking my inhaler from two puffs in the morning to one puff in the morning to every other day. He said to me, "Why don't you try to go without it now?" He said my blood tests were good.

My asthma doctor would tell me, "No matter what you do, do not stop taking your medicine." So I was afraid not to take it. The osteopath told me that I had weaned myself down, so I stopped taking it right that minute and I never went back.

How long ago was that?

About a year now.

What recommendations do you have for adults with chronic asthma or for parents with children who have asthma?

The problem with Tom Tam is he is local to the Boston area. I would tell someone to call his office and see if he can recommend someone in their local area. He also has a television station where you can watch his classes and receive energy as well. I have learned about so many of the side effects of this asthma medicine I was taking. It affects your bones. I have a dry mouth still from this medication. I would really recommend that parents look into Eastern medicine for their kids.

Did you change your diet at all to help heal your asthma?

No. I did not change it all.

Is this treatment special to Tom Tam or is this an Eastern medicine practice?

This is something he has developed. He is originally from China. He has just been phenomenal. He gives people who are really ill comfort and support. There are medical doctors that go to this. Every time I

go, there is a medical doctor with cancer sitting in the front row —
that ought to tell you something.

**Does he address every person in the room in these energy
healing classes?**

Yes. But very rarely does someone talk about asthma, because the
problems he handles are so much bigger than asthma.

**What is the difference between these energy-healing classes and
the actual personalized acupuncture sessions received?**

I think they are similar. I did energy healing and the acupuncture as a
double-prong approach to heal my asthma. If I had to choose
between the two, I would go to the energy-healing classes. You do
have to pay for the acupuncture, and the energy classes are by
donation.

**Do you say that because the energy work is less expensive, or
because you believe it to be more beneficial?**

I believe the energy-healing classes have a little bit stronger of an
impact. I am learning more about energy as I get older, and I will tell
you: there is a lot out there.

How long are these energy-healing classes?

He whips through them. You have to sit there while he talks to
everyone. The classes are about an hour and a half long. He talks to
everyone. He has a class at Spaulding Rehabilitation Hospital in
Boston. He has presented to Brown University. He presented to a
100 or so doctors and nurses at Massachusetts General Hospital. He
is definitely out-of-the-box, but I can tell you he is absolutely
amazing.

Have you talked to any other Western doctors about Tom Tam's treatment?

No, but I will tell you that I had a dear friend who passed away from a cancer no one has ever seen. He went to one of the top doctors at Brigham and Women's Hospital in Boston, and this doctor said that they refer patients to Tom Tam. I think Tom Tam and Western doctors can work hand in hand. There are things that Western doctors can do that Tom Tam can't, but I tell you what — if I was diagnosed with cancer, I would go to Tom Tam first.

...

More about Sheila: www.troublethedog.net.

#8 Diet Changes, Essential Oils & Chiropractics Cures Asthma

AnnaLaura was dependent on inhalers and steroids for controlling her asthma for the vast majority of her life. As an adult, AnnaLaura happened upon essential oils, and later made additional changes to her diet and lifestyle. The result? AnnaLaura has not needed to use her inhaler in the last five years.

Here is a bit of her story.

When were you diagnosed with asthma?

I had asthma problems my whole life. I was probably 10 or so when I was diagnosed. I could not do any kind of running, walking or hiking because of it. It would get bad, as in, I-almost-would-pass-out bad. I was on inhalers for quite a bit of time. I had allergies as well, and that would make things worse. My dad has asthma and so do some of my brothers. It runs in the family. Four or five months of the year, I had a cough. I would get a cold or something and then two, three, four months later, the cough would still be there. The doctors would just tell me to use my inhalers.

What was the treatment you were given when diagnosed?

Inhalers and allergy medicine. They thought the asthma was exercise-induced. I was told not to do a lot of strenuous exercise.

How did you ultimately cure yourself?

There were a couple of things I did. I met a woman that was selling essential oils. They had a blend called "Breathe." At the time I met her, I was annoyed with having to use inhalers. I started using the oils and noticed a difference almost immediately.

I changed my diet, too. I am allergic to wheat. I do not have celiac disease, but I try to avoid wheat. It really aggravates my asthma if I eat too much of it. Cow's milk really had a bad impact on my asthma. I started exercising more. Over time, I could do more walking and swimming. I can run more now and not have the symptoms I had before. If I start coughing, I use a little eucalyptus oil, and the cough goes away.

About a year ago, I had back pain and started going to the chiropractor. My chiropractor decided to become a chiropractor because his mom had severe asthma, and a chiropractor really helped her. Then it occurred to me that the chiropractor had done wonders for my asthma as well. So it was a culmination of a lot of things.

How do you use the oils?

The eucalyptus is not meant to be ingested, so I rub that on my neck, inhale it and put it on my chest. The peppermint you can ingest. I put that in water and drink it. It depends on the oil. The allergy oil is a peppermint-lavender blend, and I drink that.

Is there a particular brand you like?

I use doTERRA. I actually now sell the oils, but I didn't for quite some time. My whole experience with these essential oils is one of the reasons I started selling them.

How do you think the chiropractor helped your asthma?

I think a lot of things contributed to my healing from asthma. I don't know exactly how the chiropractor helped, but I think he helped in putting my whole body back into alignment.

What recommendations do you have for others who have suffered with asthma their whole lives?

The first thing I would suggest is to try essential oils. I would find a good chiropractor you can trust. I had a hard time finding a good one. See what different chiropractors have to say about asthma. You could also try a naturopathic doctor. The Western medical doctors are really limited with how they can treat you; it is just steroids and inhalers with them. Your diet is really important. What you put into your body has a big impact in you. I try to be careful with sugar. I have not eliminated a ton of sugar. I am a bit of a chocolate addict. It has really been not eating wheat and cow's milk. Cow's milk does cause a lot of breathing problems in a lot of people.

What was it like being a kid with asthma?

I live in Utah. It is beautiful, but the mountains trap a lot of the pollution. I would have a lot of days when I would have to stay indoors because the pollution levels were so high, it would affect my asthma. I would also have to stay inside when kids were playing or out at recess.

...

More about AnnaLaura: www.AnnaLauraBrown.com

#9 Cured Asthma with Homeopathy at the Age of 14

Chelsea Jones was diagnosed with asthma at the age of two. When she was 12, her mother started searching for alternative means to not just mask the symptoms of asthma, as the medicine she was prescribed for the last 10 years had, but heal her from asthma completely. Two years after beginning homeopathic treatments, Chelsea was cured.

Here is a bit of her story.

Do you have any idea what brought on your asthma at the age of two?

Yes. What my mom figured out is with a lot of kids, some kind of trauma can weaken the body and asthma-type symptoms can appear. In that regard, at that time, we had just moved and my younger sister was born. Those were two major things that happened for a young two-year-old. My mom noticed one day in my crib that I could barely breathe, and that is when I got diagnosed.

What was the treatment you were given initially?

I was put on a nebulizer. I had that for extreme circumstances, and then I had a puffer, an inhaler, for general use. The doctor recommended that my mom give me the inhaler every day, but she did not like that, so she gave it to me as needed.

How did your asthma treatment change between the ages of two and 12?

My mom started to research more and look into more of the alternative medicines. She took me off of the nebulizer, and I would only use the inhaler in a very extreme case. I would not be able to go outside in the winter if my breathing was getting short. We noticed that drinking milk would trigger asthma symptoms. I pretty much did not have any dairy.

When did homeopathy come into all of this?

It was around the age of 12 when my mom really started to try different remedies. The good thing about homeopathy is that if you try the wrong one, it won't hurt you. It just won't help you. My mom finally came across a doctor in Ottawa named Rudolf Verspoor. He had done a lot of research into sequential treatment of homeopathy. He talked to my mom about the various traumas and things that happened throughout my life, and he healed those things going backward in time. He healed those with different homeopathic remedies.

When you say traumas, does that mean emotional traumas, physical traumas — all traumas?

I think he classifies all traumas as trauma. Anything that stood out that could have affected me as a young child. As I was saying, moving and having a younger sister who was born may have triggered it. I guess that does not sound like a trauma, but it is something emotional that happens in a young kid's life.

It took two years of homeopathy to cure you of asthma?

Yes. It was about two years. For two years, leading up to being 14, my mom was giving me homeopathics basically every morning. The doctor said that there was going to be a major healing reaction in which everything would come out of me, and that would happen for a couple days. When that happened, that was the catalyst of going from being asthmatic to not being asthmatic. I do not remember it really well. I just remember getting really sick. Everything was coming out of me. After that point I never had tight breathing and basically everything that was related to asthma was not there anymore.

When you got really sick, what kind of sick was it?

I would relate it to the flu. My body got feverish and there was a lot of mucus.

Were you doing anything else to help your asthma, aside from the homeopathy?

I would go to the chiropractor every so often. A lot of people in my family would go to the chiropractor, so I guess that was just a part of our lifestyle. If I had a lot of sugar, sometimes that would weaken my immune system and trigger a cold or asthma. Keeping a simple, healthy diet went hand in hand with helping alleviate asthma symptoms.

When you finally had the healing reaction and got sick, how long were you sick?

I think it was for about four days.

Do you carry an inhaler with you now?

No.

Do you know anyone else with a story similar to yours?

I had a few friends in high school who were using their inhalers. When I try to explain how I healed myself from asthma, often people are not open to hearing it. Most people I knew that had asthma still have it and still have their inhalers.

Did you feel like your asthma was improving during these two years of taking homeopathic medicine, or did you get sick for those few days and then that was the first time you felt better?

It did not seem like anything was happening, but I think the doctor had explained to my mom that there would be a healing reaction when I would get sick, and that was what we expected. I don't think we were expecting anything until that point.

Getting sick was the healing moment. Before that, I would still have the tight chest at times and have to use the inhaler. Oftentimes, we would try not to use the inhaler. Sometimes, if people drink a bit of coffee, it helps to not have to use the inhalers. There are little things you can use when you feel an asthmatic episode going on.

Do you have any other thoughts on what you can use if people feel they are about to have an asthmatic episode?

As a preventative measure, staying hydrated helps overall. Also, dust in the air, pollens and other allergens can trigger asthmatic episodes, so keep your home clean, have the air ducts cleaned and try living somewhere with clean air if possible. Once an asthmatic episode starts, staying calm, trying to breathe slowly, and resting and having some water and a bit of caffeine can help.

What is it like being a kid with asthma?

I have three sisters, and they were all healthy. I would get made fun of a lot when I had the mask on or was using the inhaler. It was frustrating to see the other kids who seemed fine, and such little things would trigger me to get sick. It was very frustrating, always having to watch what I ate. I couldn't have ice cream at a birthday party, or that sort of thing. I played soccer as a kid. Generally, if I was feeling healthy I was OK, but at other times if I felt my immune system was weak, it would affect my ability to breathe while running.

Anything else you would like to add?

I think people should not just accept asthma. The inhaler is just masking it and not getting you anywhere. With homeopathy, there is not a one-size-fits-all solution. What worked for me may not work for everyone, but maybe a combination of many things would help. It is a journey to figure it all out.

...

To learn more about Chelsea: www.cielbleufootwear.com.

#10 Quit Asthma Inhalers Cold Turkey

Julie was diagnosed with asthma in her 20s. For almost a decade, she was dependent on inhalers. Then she met an allergist who helped her quit using her inhalers cold turkey. Julie has not used an inhaler in more than three years.

Here is a bit of her story.

What do you believe triggered getting asthma in your 20s?

Looking back, it was probably partially stress. I was in a phase in my life where I just did not know what to do yet.

Do you believe there was anything else that contributed to your getting asthma as an adult?

The only other thing I can think of is that I had a cat at the time, but I had had cats since I was about 12.

What was the treatment you were originally prescribed?

I was given an inhaler.

How long did you use your inhaler before you decided you wanted to try an alternative approach to heal your asthma?

I think in the first few years, I tried two or three different inhalers. I found an allergist, Dr. James Wolfe at Allergy & Asthma Associates of Northern California, I really liked, and he got me on an inhaler that worked for me. Then I moved to England for about seven years. The inhaler I had in America wasn't available in England, so I had to get a different one again.

It was not until I moved back from England that I went back to the allergist. He put me on a really low-dose inhaler. When you are taking all of this stuff, you become dependent on it. He got me on the lowest dose possible. Then I got pregnant, and I continued with the really low-dose inhaler. After I gave birth, I went in and he said, "We are going to take you off all the medication." I was happy, but I was afraid. The inhaler becomes a crutch. I have been totally fine for three years.

What triggered the doctor to say you could come off the inhaler?

I think he could sense and tell from the tests my asthma was not too bad. Before I went to England, he said, "One day we are going to cure you off this thing." And I just thought, "How is he going to do that?" But when he told me I should get off of it, I trusted him and he was right. I was lucky because I had a mild case of asthma. He pushed me over the edge. I trusted him.

What do you mean by your asthma being mild?

I never had an asthma attack. It was well-controlled.

How often would you use your rescue inhaler?

Maybe once or twice a month.

Was your allergist's plan to put you on the low-dose inhaler to get you off the inhalers all together?

Yes, I think it was his way of taking baby steps. At first, I was using it in the morning and at night. And then he said, "Let's just do morning," and then he said, "Let's just take you off it." And I was like, "OK, if you say so."

Did he give you a back-up inhaler just in case after he told you to stop using the inhalers all together?

Yes, he gave me a rescue inhaler, which I think I used once maybe.

It was cold turkey. Kind of like quitting smoking?

Yes, it was cold turkey. It was a little scary, but I trusted him. He was a great doctor. I knew he knew what he was talking about. I am so happy he pushed me in that direction. Like I said, the inhaler becomes a crutch and makes you feel sicker than you are.

What do you mean by that?

I would panic a little bit if I was out or at a friend's house and I didn't have my inhaler. I think that once you are given any habitual medication, the underlying message, maybe subconsciously, is "I am sick." You think that the only way you can live a normal life is because you have this "thing," and instead of focusing on healing yourself and feeling well, you form an obsession over this "thing" in your purse — as if you need it to function on a daily basis and to be without it is the worst thing that could happen to you. When actually, as evidenced by my more than three years without medication, I didn't need it!

Were there any dietary recommendations your doctor gave you?

No.

Were there any exercises you were supposed to do?

There were not. Like I was saying, the asthma and the medicine makes you feel like an invalid. It gives you an excuse not to do exercise as much or as often because, "It might trigger my asthma."

What about advice for other people who have asthma? How would you recommend they approach this?

Some of the things I wish I had looked into were breathing exercises and more alternative medicine. It did not even occur to me to look into those. Here I was, young and active, and then all of the sudden, I have these inhalers. It made me feel like I was sick.

I would also say, don't let it become a thing to you. Don't let it block what you want to do. If you find a doctor you don't like, go find one you do. I have been asthma-free for several years. My doctor was more interested in curing me than making money off of me.

...

#11 Cured Asthma with Antibiotics

At the age of 14, Ismael Navarro Jr. developed asthma symptoms literally overnight. With the help of traditional asthma-inhaler medication, Ismael's symptoms subsided significantly until the age of 25, when they came back in full force. Tired of spending hundreds of dollars on Advair every month — and even more tired of the relentless toll asthma was taking on his body — Ismael sought out a doctor who would prescribe him antibiotics in the hope that he could cure his asthma in a manner in which many others had in the past. Today Ismael lives without any asthma symptoms.

Here is a bit of his story.

You started your journey to curing yourself with antibiotics in October 2011. Your asthma symptoms were gone by February 2012. It is now July 2012. How are you doing?

I am doing well right now. I did have a sinus infection in May or June of this year. I noticed my asthma symptoms were coming back. They were not severe, but they were there. I went to the doctor and he prescribed me the Z-Pak, a five-day antibiotic treatment. I took it, and my asthma symptoms and my sinus infection went away.

Can you walk me through your journey with asthma since being diagnosed at the age of 14 to now at the age of 32?

When I was 14, I did not know what I had, but I was wheezing and I couldn't breathe. I had shortness of breath. No one in my family ever had these symptoms. I got the symptoms on a Friday evening. I went to the doctor the next day. He gave me a few puffs of Proventil, and two seconds later, I was fine. I was surprised something so simple could have helped me so much.

From being a teenager to being 25 years old, I had asthma maybe once a year, if that. But then I got it at 25 and it came back hard. I was in Arizona at the time. I tried to deal with it. I took Advair. I started looking at asthmastory.com. I had seen this website two years prior. At the time, I did not really take it seriously. The doctors just kept telling me there was not a cure for asthma. I just figured I would have asthma for the rest of my life, and I would have to deal with it. I finally decided to print off all of the information from the website and go to a doctor and ask him for the antibiotics.

My main concern I wanted to talk about with the doctor was if there would be any side effects to taking the antibiotics. He told me there would not be. He kind of tried to scare me away from taking them. He told me they would not cure my asthma, but he went ahead and gave me the prescription.

I took azithromycin in 600 milligram tablets, one daily for three days, and then one weekly for 12 weeks as recommended. There are two ways to take it. You can take a higher dosage of the pill once a week, or you can take a lower dosage more than once a week. I chose the once-a-week option because I am not good at remembering when to take meds. I noticed about a month into taking the medication that my asthma was slowly going away. I took the antibiotics for the required time, about four months. At the time that I finished the antibiotics, I was using my inhaler once a week or a couple times a week for a few weeks, but a couple of weeks after that, I was not using the inhaler at all. At first, I always had an inhaler in case there was an emergency, but since I recovered from a sinus infection, I have not used it.

During the time you had the sinus infection; did you have to use your inhaler?

Yes, I did a bit, but nothing like how I was using it prior the antibiotics treatment. I was using the emergency inhaler once an hour before I started with the antibiotics, which is not how often you are supposed to use it. When I had the sinus infection, I was using the inhaler once a day or every other day. I tried to stick out my asthma symptoms while I had the sinus infection, but it got pretty bad. I think the sinus infection triggered the asthma. I am not a doctor. I don't know, but I did get better with the Z-Pak, and I have not had asthma symptoms since and I have not used my inhaler.

Did you have health insurance when you went to the doctor for antibiotics?

No. I have not had health insurance since I was 25. I am 32 now. It is too expensive for me. Up until then, I was paying $200 to $300 a month for the Advair.

What was the cost of going to the doctor and getting the antibiotics?

The doctor visit was $80. The antibiotics were $60 to $80 total.

All the antibiotics you needed were $60 to $80?

Yes, and I am good now. It is almost like I never had asthma.

You cured asthma for $160?

Exactly. I made a video about my experience because I wanted to give people my perspective and tell people what worked for me.

When you were taking the antibiotics, were you still taking your asthma medicine daily?

Yes. I still had the asthma symptoms. But I tried to limit myself with the inhaler to see if the antibiotics were working. When I started the antibiotics, I was using my Proventil emergency inhaler every hour. Getting into the treatment, I started backing off of it, and I was only using it every couple of hours. Then I was only using it twice a day, and from there, the gap got bigger. I got to using it once a day. Then after that, I was using it once a week or twice a week, but as the weeks progressed, it got to the point where I was not using it at all.

Do you consider yourself cured?

I don't have asthmatic symptoms. I don't feel like I have it anymore. My whole life they told me there was not a cure, but I don't have any symptoms now. I will leave it to you to decide.

Do you feel comfortable leaving the house without your inhaler?

Oh, yeah. I don't carry it at all. I don't have it with me now. I have one at my house. To give you an idea, I work about 50 miles from my house. If I had an attack, I would have to drive 50 miles. I am that confident that I am not going to have an asthma attack.

Have you talked to that doctor since then about the impact the antibiotics had on your asthma?

I have not, but I will definitely be letting him know.

Do you have any idea where you picked this bacteria up from?

I have no idea.

Do you have advice for other people with asthma who are perhaps where you were before starting to take the antibiotics in October 2011?

Curing asthma gave me a different perspective on medicine and doctors. There are alternatives to dealing with disease. Whether it is asthma or anything else, the doctors are only going to tell you what they know and what they have been told to say, and it is up to the person to look for alternatives. You need to take the initiative. If whatever the doctor is giving you is not working, there are alternatives. Take that step and see what is out there. You never know until you try. Give it a shot and see if it works. Doing so was probably the best decision I ever made.

...

More about Ismael:
http://www.youtube.com/watch?v=BcfwUmZpHb4

#12 Cured Asthma with Chiropractics

Up to the age of 22, Dr. Dov Phillips would not know a life without asthma. It was not until he entered chiropractic college in New Zealand that a friend and colleague would introduce him to a technique, Network Spinal Analysis (NSA), which would ultimately cure him. Twenty or so treatments later, Dr. Phillips threw his inhalers away and has never needed them since.

Here is a bit of his story.

Can you give me an idea of what it was like to live with asthma for the first 22 years of your life?

When I was 18 months old, my mom looked down on me and saw that I was a little bit blue in the face. She took me to the hospital, and I was on preventative asthma medication pretty much from then on. I remember being a kid and not wanting to have asthma. I always heard that people grew out of it. I was taking three kinds of medicine every day, so much so that I did not really feel like I had asthma. So around my teens or late teens, I decided that as I did not have any asthma symptoms, I would go without the medicine, but the symptoms would come back and I would have to go back on the medication.

I went to Israel for a year, and with the dry climate there, my asthma went away. I was stoked. But when I came back to New Zealand, the symptoms came back after a couple of weeks. They slowly got worse, and I was back on the preventative asthma medication. I started studying pharmacology at Auckland University, so through that I was asking and learning about all the different asthma drugs available to me.

After pharmacology, my next degree was in chiropractic medicine. I asked my practitioner if he'd ever helped anyone with asthma. He started adjusting me using a technique called NSA, Network Spinal Analysis, and I started to notice improvements. I started noticing more space in my lungs. These improvements would not last long, but they were still an impressive shift. I was really impressed with NSA. I decided to have more sessions, and after a while, I started to realize my asthma had pretty much gone away.

What does NSA involve?

It is an amazing technique that involves little touches and contacts around the neck and spine. It cues the brain to find where you are storing tension and to release it.

People have two waves. One is called a somatopsychic psychic wave or body mind wave, and the other is a respiratory wave. I am sure as we sit here and are talking that you can feel tension in parts of your body. If an asthmatic has that tension around their spine or ribs, and if you can release it through NSA, it will help them breathe better.

How many NSA sessions did it take before you were no longer reliant on your inhaler?

After about eight sessions, I started noticing a big difference. Then, probably after about 20 sessions, I was fairly confident I would not need my medication anymore and went off it, but it was not that easy.

Why wasn't it easy to get off your medication?

It was a really, really hard process. My asthma was pretty much gone, but there were times I would get symptomatic again. I would get tightness in the chest. I was wondering if this was actually asthma or if this was my body's old pattern, and I would try to fight it. If the symptoms happened at night and I was lying in bed, and if I would determine I could work through it, then often I could break through. Sometimes, if I was really tired, I would take my inhaler and I would feel instantly better, but then the next day, almost 18 hours after I had taken my inhaler, my asthma would come back. On the days and nights where I could break through without using my inhaler, I would be fine for a long time afterwards, but on the days or nights where I used the inhaler, almost exactly 18 hours later, I would start having the symptoms again.

One thing I started to notice that was really interesting was the thing that was triggering those symptoms were advertisements on TV for asthma medications or seeing a kid on TV with asthma. Somehow, it would trigger something in me, and that night I would have problems breathing. That went on for about three months.

When was the last time you used your inhaler?

About nine years ago. I have since thrown them all out. I have not had them for so long. It is not even a part of my consciousness anymore.

Do you as a doctor have advice on how or where people should start on the journey of curing themselves of asthma?

Just start. I don't think it really matters as long as you have started. There are so many things that will help, and doing one thing that is positive is way better than doing nothing. What works for one person will not necessarily work for another. I like the natural approach, personally. The answer to this question is a bit complicated, as it depends on what triggers a person's asthma and why they have it. Along with the physical triggers, it has also been shown that there is a huge correlation between emotions and asthma.

How so?

There are a lot of studies that show an emotional event can trigger asthma, and that makes sense to me. There is a theory regarding the idea that when you are breathing well, there is a message to and from the brain coming from the proprioceptors sensory receptors in the costovertebral joint (where the rib head meets the spine) indicating that you are breathing well. And if for some reason there is no movement, no stimulation, the message is no longer present and it, if you will, sends alarm bells off and you feel like you are not breathing well. Sometimes asthmatics feel they are not breathing well or not getting enough oxygen, and then they have that panicked or tight feeling.

However, they have done studies to show that these asthmatics are in actuality really well-oxygenated or at times over-oxygenated when they are experiencing this feeling of tightness. The thought is that it's not that they aren't getting enough oxygen, but that there is a perception they are not getting enough oxygen based on the ribs not moving well. When the joints connecting the spine and ribs are not working as they should be, and the brain is not getting the message that they are breathing well, the response is that the brain incorrectly thinks, "I am not breathing."

In my experience, the fact that there is a cures for asthma is not being widely communicated in the United States or Spain. Is this the case in New Zealand and if so, why do you think that is?

Everyone knows chiropractors are not really always respected in the traditional Western medical realm. When I was going into chiropractic college, my dad asked a family friend who is an internationally respected medical doctor what he thought of chiropractors. His response was, "I see they have a place when they talk about backs, but when they talk about things like asthma, it really pisses me off." He hated it that we "alternative medicine quacks" would go around and talk about how we could cure asthma. It really pissed him off. I have always found that very funny because that has been my experience in how Western medicine reacts to chiropractors and our helping asthmatics. It's also funny because for me, it's changed my life.

Why do you think this is Western medicine's reaction?

There are so many factors. In medical school, there are so many things to learn that students cannot possibly learn everything. Everything is evidence-based with Western medicine. If it is not evidence-based, then it could not possibly be true or real. With chiropractic, you have a percentage of people who have amazing results and other people who don't, so Western medicine writes it off to the placebo effect or as anecdotal, and they negate it. I think that is partly because of who they are or what their training makes them do.

What I do not understand is that there are a number of people who are curing themselves of asthma. At what point do you think these people who are now cured will be considered evidence to the fact that there could be a cure?

There has to be enough evidence that is also reproducible. This means that pretty much everyone needs to get the same response or at least the majority needs to get that response. But it still comes down to beliefs, and if you don't believe a therapy will work as a doctor, you won't prescribe it to your patient.

Is the same not true with Western medical approaches in regard to medications and practices that work for some, but do not necessarily work for everyone?

Great point. In fact, all drugs are tested and compared to placebos, and they have to be more effective than the placebo. Often the amount by which they are different is not that much. What I find interesting is that the placebo works on every condition for a percentage of the focus group, whereas the drug they are testing only works for that one condition.

On a slightly different note: if you look at cancer treatments, you will see that lots of treatments only work short-term, and obviously not for everyone and not all the time.

If someone is on the journey to curing asthma, when or how would they know that going to a chiropractor would be helpful?

There are so many beneficial reasons to go to a chiropractor, as long as you go to someone who is interested in really helping you. You need to go to someone whose heart is in the right place, as is the case with anything.

If you are aware that when you are having asthmatic symptoms you have a lot of tightness around your neck, upper back and shoulders, and if you feel that tightness first and then you have the asthmatic reaction, going to a chiropractor could be enormously helpful. If your asthma is triggered around stressful or emotional times, then the NSA approach would be ideal. I think some people do not realize that stress is triggering their asthma because stress is such a part of their lives that they are not even entirely aware of it. They think their asthma, which is really being triggered by stress, is coming out of nowhere.

Did you change your diet to help your asthma?

In my transition time, if I had too many refined carbohydrates, too much Coke, white bread or refined, sugary foods, I would get asthmatic or more into that wheezy place. As a kid, I had a lot of refined carbohydrates and I think that played a huge, huge part in my asthma.

Did you try any other alternative techniques in healing your asthma, or was NSA the first?

NSA was the first.

What advice do you have as a chiropractor and someone who had asthma for other asthmatics?

Look at your diet. That is something you can change straightaway. Again, it depends on the individual. Is it a kid? Is it someone who developed asthma late in life? Is it env¬ironmental?

As an aside, I also find it weird that when kids have a tight chest and go to the doctor, the doctor tells them they have asthma and from that point on, they think have asthma even though they might not. They just had symptoms similar to asthmatic symptoms, and now think they need they need asthma medicine when in reality they never had it. Just like me: I can guarantee you that after not taking the inhaler for years, if I took it tonight, my body would think I would need it tomorrow in 18 hours.

But general advice I would give is: go away from refined carbohydrates. Drink less milk and eat less dairy, which is a common trigger. Go get your spine checked, and be open-minded about it. Give it a few sessions, and see if it works. Don't expect it to change straightaway, because it won't. But see if there is a noticeable difference. It does not work for everyone but when it works, it works 100 percent for you.

How have you helped other asthmatics?

I have never had a person go completely off of his or her asthma medication, and I think that's because so many people get to the point of needing to make the conscious decision of no longer being an asthmatic. There are those few nights in which they have to push through — and you have to be willing to push through — and they are not willing to do that. I have probably worked with about 15 asthmatics, and I think every single one except for one has reduced their medication significantly. I have not had any miracle stories yet.

You are your miracle story.

Yes, I am. I think there is only one person I have not helped at all, but with most people it is a huge shift with a massive reduction in medication.

Tell me about the process of pushing through it. How did you do it? Do you have advice for others?

Be very careful doing it, because you are putting yourself in a state that is very challenging. Only do it if you are already strong and healthy. If you have something else health-wise going on, it might not be the right thing for you to do. If you have cardiovascular disease or have had a stroke, then it is not for you. Anyone in their 30s or younger who is in good health and without other issues will, I believe, adapt.

The process involves deciding that you may not actually be asthmatic, but you are having symptoms that are similar to asthmatic symptoms and your body can adapt. It is keeping focused on that idea.

I became aware that there are two trigger points on your trapezius muscle. If you push down on it with both hands, you can get an increase in breath. I have tested it with other asthmatics, and it seems to provide temporary relief.

If you are going to go back to the drugs, it is quite hard to break free. If you fall off and start taking the medicine again, just start trying to break through again. If I had given up after the sixth try, I would still be on the medication today.

I am interested in your thoughts on having asthma as a part of your identity.

That is the whole thing: the struggle with the old sense of self, the one who was the asthmatic and needed the inhaler. The ego defines itself by who you are and who you were. When you say, "I am an asthmatic," that is who you are. You are linking yourself with that disease and experience. Why is it that you link yourself to it?

Asthmatics think, "If I am an asthmatic and if asthmatics have this experience, that means that I have this experience." It comes down to asking yourself, "Can I choose a different experience in life?"

When I would unconsciously see those adverts, it would trigger that asthmatic response in me. The adverts were, "Are you an asthmatic? Do you have problems breathing?" And even though I had not had problems in weeks or months, all of the sudden, those symptoms would come back.

Is there anything else you would like to add?

Drugs are going to give you temporary relief. Your life is probably not going to get better by taking them. Be grateful that they have probably saved your life. If you need to fall back on them, that is OK, but then try something else. Be open-minded to the possibility that you could live a life without it. There are so many things out there that could help you. Go for it. Just go for it. It is worth it.

…

More about Dr. Phillips: www.inspiringwellness.co.nz.

#13 Cured Asthma on Day Three of a Seven-Day Cleanse

Karen was diagnosed with asthma around the age of 35. Her asthma started with severe allergies that were triggered when she moved into her fiancé's house in February 2000. Within a year, she was having asthma attacks every night at 3 a.m. She tried numerous therapies and remedies to heal herself, then she tried a fast. On the third day of the fast, her asthma stopped. She has not had any asthma symptoms since.

Here is a bit of her story.

What remedies did you use to try to cure yourself?

I tried hot and cold showers, drinking warm broth, a neti pot for nasal irrigation, massage, infrared saunas, pulling up old carpeting, doing coffee enemas and cleaning radiators like my life depended on it.

My husband's house was an old German Tudor. We had it tested for mold and the results came back so minimal that it couldn't have been the issue. I do believe it had something to do with the very old carpeting we had in that house. We did remove it from the bedroom, which helped, but we never did remove it from the living room or dining room.

Did you find that any of those treatments significantly helped you in alleviating asthma symptoms?

Yes, the hot and cold showers did help with congestion and so did cleaning up my environment. There's this stigma around things like coffee enemas, however, they made such a huge difference as far as my congestion. It was amazing.

What do you believe ultimately cured you?

I did a seven-day fast following the book The Tao of Health, Sex & Longevity. The asthma stopped on Day Three and has never come back. I healed my allergies with liver cleansing.

What liver cleanse did you do?

I healed my allergies with liver cleansing based on the Hulda Clark protocol. I did about 11 liver cleanses over the next two years and eliminated all allergies.

When was the last time you used your inhaler or any asthma medication?

2001.

Did you make changes to your diet to cure your asthma?

Now I eat a very low-carbohydrate diet, but back then, I still ate carbohydrates. I ate pretty clean and mostly vegetarian. I ate lentils and chapati. It was the fast that cured me, and I continued doing small fasts and eating cleanses afterward.

Did you continue doing the fasts and cleanses to stave off asthma symptoms or were these for general health purposes?

I did for a few years, however, now I follow the Primal Blueprint diet. It isn't a diet that I found and began doing, but one that my body led me to. I do not eat any grains or legumes at all. A very low carb diet resonates with my body. Everybody is different, and this is what my body likes.

Did you integrate any particular exercises into your lifestyle to assist yourself in curing asthma?

Yoga, but it was hard because I was often congested. I would go running too, but not as faithfully as I once did.

Did you integrate any additional treatments such as massage therapy, acupuncture, chiropractic or any other therapies in curing yourself?

Yes, massage, chiropractic, Emotional Freedom Technique/tapping and acupuncture.

Did you find any of these treatments did or did not help in curing your asthma?

None truly gave me relief. Massage was nice for relaxation, but all I cared about was being able to breathe.

What mistakes do you believe people with asthma make in handling their asthma?

Some people do not understand the relationship between the health of their colon and their ability to breathe.

Could you explain a little more of what you mean regarding the relationship between the health of the colon and a person's ability to breathe?

Well, I am no expert. I am simply someone who has some real life experience. In my case, as soon as I did a coffee enema, I could breathe. There has to be something to that. If there are toxins backed up in your system, then your body can't do its job of keeping the place clean and efficient. Also, it is common for yogis to do enemas to deepen their breathing during yoga. It is hard to argue with 2000 years of wisdom.

What advice do you have for someone who would like to begin the journey of healing or curing their asthma?

Do a detox any way you can. There are slow and fast options. Cleanse the colon.

Did you integrate any supplements, tonics, potions, antibiotics and/or essential oils into your life to help cure asthma?

For supplements I took a lot of vitamin C, Methyl Sulfonyl Methane (MSM). and colloidal silver and did steam treatments. I did the steam treatments from the stove, not the kind you get from the doctor. I also did Chinese herbs and had an inhaler as well. I asked my doctor if there was anything I could be doing naturally or with food to help with my asthma and her response was, "If you are not going to take the meds, don't waste my time writing the prescription." This is what spurred my mission to heal myself.

...

#14 Doctor Cured His Asthma Holistically

Dr. Richard Firshein was diagnosed with asthma as a child. As very few asthma treatments existed at the time, his asthma symptoms were managed by, as he says, "staying indoors, taking the few medications available and suffering." By his late 20s, he had finished medical school. He was teaching and directing a residency program. Then one morning, he awoke completely unable to breathe. The diagnosis he received while in intensive care was grim. Although doctors were unsure if he would make it, he knew he had the tools to survive. Once released from the hospital, Dr. Firshein spent a year weaning himself off eight different asthma medications and creating a program that would not only ultimately cure him of asthma, but help heal his asthma patients and asthmatic children in a local Bronx school.

Here is a bit of his story.

Tell me what transpired after you left the hospital.

Prior to going to the hospital, I had been studying different breathing techniques, reading research, studying diets and different supplements for asthma, but there was not a cohesive program available.

Once I finally got through that time in the hospital, I spent the next year weaning myself off about eight different medicines. I set a course to find alternative treatments other than those that were currently available. I started to incorporate what I found for myself into my practice with my asthmatic patients. I was having incredible successes, to the point where people were getting off their asthma medication and living much fuller lives. Asthma is a very complicated problem, but one where there are natural solutions available.

Much in the way that others went around thinking about heart disease, I thought about asthma. I thought about how diet and lifestyle could impact asthmatics lives. Over the course of several years of successes with myself and other asthmatics, I wrote my first book, Reversing Asthma, and a second book, Your Asthma-Free Child.

You did a program with kids with high asthma rates in a school in the Bronx as well.

Prior to writing my second book, I incorporated all of the techniques I had learned and created my Breath of Life program. I incorporated this program into my practice as well, but I wanted to test it. I selected one of the schools with the highest rates of asthmatic children, which just happened to be in the Bronx.

From this school I took the kids with the worst attendance and hospitalization records or any other problem I could find that was on the top of the scale, and I started my Breath of Life program with them. We had incredible success and results.

Kids with the worst attendance went to having the best attendance records. Kids with asthma started helping their parents with asthma. We were keeping people out of the emergency room. There were all kinds of wonderful successes.

What were the components of the program you tested with the children?

The mainstays of the program were to first look at their environment and get very serious about making sure anything they were potentially allergic to was removed, such as dust or dust mites. If they were exposed to radon or asbestos or anything toxic in their home, I made sure that was removed.

Then we looked at their diet. I substituted omega-3 fatty acids for trans fats. I made sure they were eating monosaturated fats instead of polysaturated fats. I incorporated more olive oil into their diet and took out butter, creams and milk products. I took out wheat from their diet. I tested them for food allergies and eliminated any allergies found. I really put together a super-clean diet for them. I had them do detox diets. I eliminated all these harmful things in their diets, and then I started looking at supplements to support them.

There were a lot of supplements that I found useful, such as magnesium and fish oils. After supplements, I then incorporated breathing exercises I had developed by working with patients. These included a combination of techniques from yoga and Ayurvedic medicine. I also incorporated other natural modalities such as visualization, meditation, hypnosis and exercise. I developed a pulse exercise to condition asthmatic lungs and muscles. More recently, I have added into my program allergy treatments and drops, as about 50 percent of the asthma patients I treat have significant allergy issues in conjunction with their asthma. All of these things encompass the entire Breath of Life program.

How are people responding to this program?

I have been doing this practice for about 20 years, specifically using these approaches and techniques. What I have found is more and more people are gravitating toward it. It is becoming something people understand. Instead of using some of the toxic drugs, people are learning how to help themselves with their own skill sets.

Treating asthma is not a simple process.

People need to understand it is a very complicated problem. I have patients who have asthma triggers from cold, from heat, dust, chlorine, toxic chemicals, perfumes and other things. It is not a simple problem. For asthmatics, it requires a very full understanding of all the things that go on. It is complicated. I believe they have discovered 20 genes that regulate asthma.

Is the approach you designed how you healed yourself?

Yes. Everything I do and everything I have done, I tested myself. I am my own guinea pig. I was very skeptical of everything. What worked with me, I would incorporate with my patients.

You talk on your website about how you were suffering needlessly as an asthmatic. Do you think most asthmatics are suffering needlessly?

I think every asthmatic is suffering needlessly. I am not saying everyone is going to be cured, but if you are not within the normal spectrum of living and if you are not enjoying your life, you are suffering needlessly.

You have talked about the side effects of the traditional asthma medication provided by Western medicine. Could you talk about that a little more?

Cortisone is a very powerful anti-inflammatory and it is used as a last-ditch effort we have to help asthmatics, but a lot of times doctors use it as a first line of treatment. Treating asthma is very complicated. With every asthmatic attack, it can take four to six weeks to recover, but people think if they take a drug and the next day they are better, then their asthma is gone.

These medications are covering up the wound, but the wound is still there. There is a way to deal with this long-term. Certainly medication can provide a bridge, but not a very effective one. Drugs like albuterol, if overused, can cause cardiac arrest. In moderation, all these things are helpful, but the way we recommend the drugs right now is not very thoughtful.

On your website, you say, "Asthma teaches us about the mysterious dialogue between mind and body." Can you talk about that a little bit?

Your body and mind have the ability to focus energy and regulate how we function. Meaning that your mind can help you overcome a certain amount of stress. If we can learn to control our mind and control our stress, then we can have a great degree of control over our asthma.

Many times, asthma is triggered in response to something in the environment. It may take a bit of time for that response to dissipate, but if your mind is not at ease, if it is anxious or panicked, whatever experience you are going through will seem much, much worse. The connection between the mind and body can be really powerful because using meditation, visual imagery and hypnosis can really train your mind to focus itself and assist in overcoming a problem like asthma.

Is there a cornerstone to your asthma program that you consider more critical than anything else?

Over the years, I have had differences of opinions. At the end of the day, it is the trifecta of diet, supplements and the environment. Those are the things you have to deal with first. The second layer, which seals the deal, is visualization, meditation, exercise and generally taking your body to the next place.

When was the last time you used your inhaler?

It has been a number of years, at least five to seven years.

How is the rate of asthma changing in the U.S.?

In 1980, there were seven to 12 million asthmatics. In 2006, there were at least 36 million asthmatics. The rate has tripled. We are dealing with an epidemic that is not controlled. Sometimes our knowledge and use of the medications we have are giving people the chance to function normally, but it would be great to take it to the next level and get people to really understand how their bodies are working and the importance of all of these techniques I talked about so we could get these numbers to reverse, to go backwards.

Anything else you would like to add?

Every condition is a warning and an opportunity. If you can treat asthma as an opportunity, then in every other aspect of your life, you will become healthier. That goes not only for asthma but any medical condition. To understand there is an opportunity within a condition to heal and to grow will not only heal the problem, but will heal the person as well.

...

More about Dr. Firshein: www.drfirshein.com.

Diagnosed with Asthma in Her 40s, Healed Herself in Her 50s

Katherine lived four decades without asthma. Shortly after moving to Atlanta from Connecticut, she started getting a tight chest when she ran in colder weather. A moldy apartment would later push her to inhaler dependence. Additional health problems caused Katherine to making significant changes to her diet and lifestyle. Today Katherine has made huge strides in healing her asthma.

Here is a bit of her story:

Tell me about how you developed asthma in your 40s.

I moved to Georgia when I was 40. I was a runner. I started running when it was cold out, and I would get this annoying tightness in my chest. I then moved to a moldy place. I would wake up and could hardly breathe. A few years later, I went to a doctor and I was diagnosed with asthma. At this point I knew I had to do something because this was not going to get any better on its own.

What was triggering your asthma?

I had my blood tested for food sensitivities and they found the usual culprits – wheat and dairy. I gave up wheat and in two and half weeks my health was a lot better.

Did you do anything else other than giving up wheat and dairy?

I read a book about reversing asthma that talked about fish oil. What I started doing was taking Nordic Naturals Fish Oil in a teaspoon. I recently changed that to a tablespoon. I take a tablespoon after breakfast. I don't think there is anything bad about having more fish oil than that, but that is what I take. You could also eat salmon, but it would have to be wild salmon. Fish is a scary thing these days because all of it is loaded with toxins. You have to take fish oil produced from wild fish. The Nordic Naturals Fish Oil is not cheap, but it is worth the price. You can't take regular fish oil capsules because you would need to take 16 capsules to get the daily dose of what you need.

I went to an allergist and had complete allergy testing, with the pin pricks. They found out that I was allergic to almost everything. I started allergy shots, which I kept up for about five years.

I have read a lot since then about getting the good fats into your diet and getting the bad fats out of your diet to improve your health. Bad fats are any of the seed oils, such as corn oil or vegetable oil. You need to also stop eating things like mayonnaise and prepared salad dressings. Now I fry or heat in coconut oil and use olive oil on "cold" food like salad. The problem with with this diet, of course, is you can't eat out at most restaurants and you can't buy processed food.

Did you make any other modifications to your diet to help your asthma?

I drive across town to get butter from cows that eat grass. I never heat olive oil because it denatures it and your body can't digest and utilize it properly. I do not eat much beef, but what I eat is grass-fed. I eat eggs from an actual farm, which are getting easier to get these days in Atlanta. I eat two eggs every day. You have to eat eggs over-easy or poached to get the benefit of the runny yolk. I don't eat potatoes, bread, breakfast cereal or pizza. I cook my meals from scratch. I eat salmon. It is hard to do this diet, but I would rather use the diet than take medicine for my asthma, as the side effects of those medications are not good for you.

I also accidentally reversed periodontal disease with this diet. Three or four years into the diet, my gums became perfect. The dentist did not want to hear that I cured this disease with diet. He looked actually angry with me when I told him I cured myself. At one point he said to me, "I don't believe you ever had problems." And I said, "Look at the charts." Sure enough, five years ago, they were measuring the gaps in my gums.

Did you make any changes to your home environment?

I got very serious about my home environment. I went out and bought covers to go over my mattresses. I took all of the carpet out of my bedroom. I change my sheets once a week so the dust mites do not get to me. I know now if I don't keep my sheets really clean I will wake up with a tight chest from the dust mites.

After making the changes to my diet and home, all of my health problems started to improve. I felt my asthma very much ease up. In 2006, I had a lot of sinus problems, and my doctor gave me nasal saline, which had a wonderful effect on opening up my nasal passages.

How often do you use your inhaler now?

I would say that I use my rescue inhaler, albuterol, two or three times a month now. The air in Atlanta is very poor in the summer, and on two occasions I had to call the doctor and take QVAR, a corticosteroid spray, to calm down the inflammation in my lungs. I am going on vacation to Guadalupe soon. The air is very clean there, and I always feel really good while I am there.

When I began this journey, I had to move out of my apartment because of the mold. I remember one time, I went to a bar and I could smell the mold and had to leave because of it. Now I can go to where I please, dance, breathe, socialize and have no tightness in my chest.

Could you talk more about good oils and the bad oils?

Commercial seed oils are bad to eat because they are refined with heat. There is a huge body of literature and a ton of controversy around this, but any of the natural healing books you pick up these days will talk about the negative impact of commercial oils. There are a lot of people who talk about the deleterious effects of these bad oils. Some good books are Nourishing Traditions and Good Fats, Bad Fats. Before World War II, we ate a lot of fat. They made pies from lard. We drank milk with milk fat. That was back in the days when cows were in fields. We ate butter from cows that actually ate grass. Those were fats that would the soothe inflammation that causes asthma. Coconut oil was very prevalent in the United States before World War II. People were accustomed to seeing it and using it. Coconut oil is a bit of a pain because it is a solid below 76 degrees, so you can't just pour it, but it actually has a very nice flavor.

Prior to World War II, seed oils were only used in paint and similar things, but the "edible oil industry," as they call themselves, found a way to refine these oils and to take the objectionable taste and odor out. When I look at that, I think, "Do I really want to eat something that was once used in paint?" The oil companies denature the seeds so much in the heating process that when these oils get into your body, your body just does not know what to do with them and as such they contribute to inflammation and probably predispose people for asthma, not to mention arterial damage.

In an email to me you said, "Asthma is a symptom of inflammation but not a disease."

If you look around at all the kids and people that have asthma, you will see people who are eating the wrong foods, the wrong oils and living in toxic environments with bad air. In other words, with a lot of those people, if you moved them where the air was clear and you gave them good food, they would probably be rid of their asthma symptoms.

Was there anything else that was important in healing your asthma?

I started drinking triple-filtered reverse-osmosis water. I go to the health-food store once a week and fill my water jars up. I remove the fluoride and chlorine from my diet by doing this. I am not a vegetarian. I think animal products are really important. If you look at the average person who shops at the supermarket, they are never eating anything that is not polluted or bad for them. It's tragic. No wonder so many people are sick.

If people eat supermarket meat — God help them. If they eat supermarket fish — God help them. The vegetables at supermarkets are sprayed with pesticides and are grown in soil without nutrients. People think they are healthy because they choose foods based on listening to advertisements from the food industry. They have a "healthy" breakfast cereal which is just a simple carbohydrate. They will have a glass of milk, and do I need to repeat the problems with the milk supply? They will have a glass of juice in the morning. All of this is toxic — it's simple carbohydrates and it has no nutrients. They will have a sandwich at lunch with lunchmeat that is loaded with preservatives. The amount of preservatives in lunch meat is ridiculous. For dinner they will have pasta or pizza. So, at the end of the day, what have they eaten? Nothing that nourishes them, and that is why people get sick.

There is a book out now called Deep Nutrition. It is about how important vegetables really are and how they do what they do in our bodies. There is a woman, Terry Wahls, who is a doctor at the University of Iowa. She had M.S. and was in a wheelchair. She was not satisfied with the answers that doctors were giving her, so she went and did her own research. Basically, by eating a ton of vegetables, she is now out of her wheelchair. She wrote a book called Minding My Mitochondria. These books are great reading if you want to inspire yourself to stick to your good-food diet.

How did you figure out what would heal your asthma?

By reading books and doing research on the Internet.

Do you attribute any one thing to curing your asthma?

You need to eat the good fats to calm the bad inflammation. You have to get rid of the bad fats, which cause the inflammation, and you have to get rid of the allergens. The cure is in food, fish oils and fats. Get very serious about cleaning up your environment and when you go on vacation, go where the air is clean.

Do you talk to your Western doctor about your approach to healing asthma?

She just looks at me and says, "Good, good for you. Very interesting." She is not a health nut. She is 50 pounds overweight. Everyone in the office is. She is interested in what I am finding out. She has a very open mind. She's the one who showed me the saline rinse for my blocked nasal passages, so I will always love her.

I go to my allergist every year for a checkup. The nurse, who is overweight, tells me that her asthma is not great, but she is keeping it under control. This last time I was there, she told me her daughter's asthma was really bad. I looked at her and said, "Stop eating wheat and start eating the right fats." And she said, "Oh, really?" I went a little bit further in describing my diet, and I just watched her eyes glaze over while she completely discounted what I was saying. Someone like this only has faith in the meds.

...

The Homeopath Who Healed Her Son of Asthma

Sara Chana's son was born with severe eczema. Then at 18 months old he was diagnosed with asthma. Western medicine offered her antibiotics, hydrocortisone and steroids to alleviate but not heal the symptoms of both. Sara refused to accept this is as a lifelong prognosis for her son. She spent countless sleepless nights researching herbs and homeopathy and in the end healed her son of both. Today she is a homeopath.

Here is a bit of their story.

Were your son's asthma and eczema related?

Lots of kids with eczema turn up with asthma but not all kids with asthma get eczema. The correlation between eczema and asthma is very strong. My son started wheezing when he was about one and a half years old. He was on a nebulizer and could barely breathe. He had allergy controlled pillow cases and bedding. I bought air filters. He did not eat any foods with chemicals in them and he was still wheezing because he had an over reactive airway. A little dust mite would get in there and his lungs would start to quiver, shake and compress in on themselves. My son still has a slight over reactive immune system but herbs and homeopathy keep it in line.

Both asthma and eczema are a hyper-reaction of the immune system. People with asthma and / or eczema have an over active immune system. When people are having a hyper-reaction their body is misreading the signals around it. The body is reading these non-toxic triggers as if they are toxic and the body, skin and/or lungs hyper-respond.

What are examples of irritants and allergens that trigger the asthmatic over reactive airway?

Hair spray, perfume, dust mites, molds, smog, tobacco smoke.

Can stress be one of the things that cause this hyper-reaction?

Everybody is stressed in this world. When somebody is stressed their weakness will come out. The person who gets migraines when put under stress will get migraines. The person who gets acne when put under stress will get acne. Stress is going to exacerbate any pre-existing condition. It is not that asthmatics are more stressed; it is just that under stress they have a propensity to have asthmatic symptoms.

Did you use one approach to heal both the eczema and the asthma in your son?

Yes. They were treated the same way. We balanced his immune system with homeopathy and we reduced the inflammation and eczema wounds with herbs. Homeopathy stimulates the body to balance itself. Herbs heal tissues and work on the internal organs. His body is no longer responding to the asthma triggers or environmental triggers which were causing the asthmatic response. He is in college now and he is functioning like a normal adult.

How long did this take for his body to stop having asthmatic symptoms?

It takes from 4 to 6 months for the body to begin to readjust itself.

Do you recommend homeopathy and herbs as a way to cure asthma?

I like to use herbs and homeopathic remedies [for asthma]. There are over 3000 homeopathic remedies available to balance the system. I do not always get it right the first time.

I like to use herbs to heal the system. I will often give a herb called Cramp Bark Herb which will stop the spasming of the lungs. I will give an herb called Elecampane that helps clean out the mucus. Often asthmatics over produce mucus and as such I give them Yerba Santa which clears the nasal passages of mucus. I give them Usnea for upper respiratory infections.

Herbs take longer than homeopathic remedies. When I get the right homeopathic remedy the person will feel better in an hour. The right homeopathic remedy goes with both the symptoms and the personality of the person, whereas with herbs I typically treat the symptoms and not the name of the disease. We don't treat the name of the disease. We treat the symptoms in homeopathy.

How does homeopathy work with adults who have chronic asthma?

There is a very interesting discussion in homeopathy when you are healing chronic illness in adults; it often follows a pattern that old illnesses reappear and disappear. A famous homeopath named Dr. Hering said that when you give the correct remedy the illness will heal from the above downwards, from within to without, from a more important organ to a less important organ in the reverse order in which you got these illnesses. We use homeopathy to unfold these illnesses backwards. Maybe as a kid a patient had mumps, then eczema and then strep throat. The body needs to untangle itself from these illnesses it had before the chronic illness developed to fully heal itself with homeopathic remedies.

Sometimes an adult will have had eczema in the cracks of their arms as a kid and then they take a homeopathic remedy and get eczema in the cracks of their arms for a few months. If an adult broke his arm as a child as he is going through the homeopathic remedies his arm may hurt for a few weeks as the body rebuilds and restructures itself.

With homeopaths we cure as much by the psyche and the emotional state of the person as we do by the disease state. People like to go to homeopaths because we take a deep interest in them.

What is the relationship between immunity issues and asthma?

Most asthmatics have a compromised immune system. They can have food induced asthma. A lot of them have viral induced asthma or exercise induced asthma. Most asthmatics ability to function in the world is not great. That is why you see in films the one kid who is getting picked on is the one kid that needs his inhaler. Asthmatics are more vulnerable to everything around them in their lives. Breathing is so vitally important that they tend to be more fearful. They are more vulnerable to germs and bugs. They tend to be more vulnerable beings.

What type of doctor should an asthmatic look for? A homeopath? A naturopath? An acupuncturist?

Breathing is life and death. If you go to an alternative practitioner and they say they are going to be able to get you off your asthma medicine in three weeks, I would leave. I never take my clients off of their asthma medicine until we build up their immune system. We go slowly. We keep them on that asthma medicine for a couple of months.

If anyone offers you a miracle drug walk out. If they want you to buy $300 of herbs walk out. I would not do acupuncture for children under 10 because needles hurt. A naturopathic doctor is a great idea but there are not a lot around. Craniosacral is fabulous, but that is with bodies and energies that are out of line and for my asthmatics they need to spend money internally. If my asthmatics have money I will send them to a craniosacral therapist. There is nothing better because they will put them back in line for the body misalignment associated with wheezing. I don't believe chiropractors should dispense herbs because most of them are not trained in herbal medicine. Herbs are not part of chiropractic training. I believe homeopathy and herbal remedies are the best for the asthmatic person, but I think craniosacral is great for asthma as well.

What is the philosophy of homeopathy?

The man who started homeopathy believes the body is meant to heal itself and I absolutely believe that. The body is a self healing mechanism and we just need to take steps to get the body to the position where it can totally function for itself. If you take steroids it stops the immune system. If you take antibiotics it stops the immune system. Asthma medicine is a Vasa dilator. It dilates the air passages, but it does not let the body do it on its own. We as homeopaths really believe the body is a self healing mechanism and we just need to help and support it.

The founder of homeopathy would say if someone comes to you with a chronic cough you can give him a great homeopathic remedy, but if he lives in a dark, moldy basement that cough is going to come back so you need to get him out of that dark moldy basement. If someone comes to me for asthma and she is in a terrible marriage and hates her job; my job as a homeopath is to get her out of that environment. My job as a homeopath is to get my patients into a healthy environment. If things are bothering you daily you will never get better. In order for your body to self-heal itself sometimes you need to change your environment.

How long was it before your son's asthma was significantly healed?

He was off the nebulizer by the time he was four years old and then only used it when he needed it. I would not say he is completely cured. He was born with a compromised immune system.

What are the long terms effects of being on the inhalers or other traditional Western pharmaceuticals for asthma control?

People become addicted to their asthma medicine. With steroids the lung tissue thins and they become resistant to the medication over time. None of my patients get addicted to herbs or homeopathic remedies.

What diet recommendations do you have for asthmatics?

I believe 100% in Dr. D'Adamo's blood type diet. I feel diet makes a huge difference in asthmatics life.

What recommendation do you have for exercise?

If you don't exercise you will not be healthy. As a homeopath I try to figure out which exercise my patient will be compliant with.

...

More about Sara: www.sarachana.com.

Chiropractor Healed Her Asthma Holistically

Dr. Katie Hawn lived asthma-free for 23 years. Then, a cat at a friend's house triggered a quick decline in her respiratory health, until she was at the point where she was hospitalized and diagnosed with asthma. Dr. Hawn, afraid of going down the path of lifelong asthmatic drug dependency, sought out her own treatment to not only suppress her asthma symptoms, but to heal them. Today, Dr. Hawn lives virtually asthma-free.

Here is a bit of her story.

You lived until you were 23 without asthma and then a cat triggered it?

That's right. When I was little I played with cats on my uncle's dairy farm every summer with no problems, but one deep breath of this particular little kitten overwhelmed my system.

Were you doing anything to treat yourself for your asthma after this, or was it just trying to stay away from cats?

At first, I just avoided cats, and that seemed to be enough. When I was exposed to cats, I might start sneezing and my nose would run, and this was frequently accompanied by asthma. Sometimes I reacted pretty badly, but not bad enough to go get an inhaler.

Years later, a good friend of mine had a cat she was caring for that I fell in love with. I knew I was allergic, but someone had told me you could get used to the dander if you had little bits of exposure. So I tried it.

But at the end of one week, I knew I was in trouble. I sequestered the cat, cleaned the house and tried all the holistic remedies I could find. I got homeopathic medicines, Chinese medicines and went to my craniosacral therapist. Although each treatment helped a little, my system was just becoming overwhelmed. Eventually, I was so tired of trying to breathe that I knew if I did not do something, I was going to die.

I went to the emergency room. The doctors took x-rays, and then gave me one round of inhaled medication. I lay there, thinking "Oh great, my lungs are ruined now because of all this junk they just pumped into them." After five hours of treatment, I finally went home to recover. After that, I got asthma with everything: exertion, cold air and with cats, of course.

How did you treat your asthma after you were hospitalized?

The first thing I did was find a therapist that was certified in a technique called NAET, or Nambudripad's Allergy Elimination Technique. Using a non-invasive diagnosis method commonly called "muscle testing," she ran me through a testing and treatment protocol, first addressing basic allergies, then soon treating for cat dander, cat hair, and the air in the house I was living in. After five treatment sessions, I tested clear for all known cat allergies. NAET helped decrease the severity of my reaction, but didn't cure the asthma completely.

A few years later, despite my best preparation, I was exposed again to cat dander in a way I couldn't quite control. I found a top-rated pulmonologist and made an appointment. He gave me a daily inhaler for morning and night, and then the other inhaler for more severe reactions. I used the inhalers as little as possible — I knew I had to have them in order to stay alive and functional, but at the same time, I actively sought out other treatments.

Why didn't you want to use the asthma drugs?

I was extremely wary of creating any kind of drug dependency. Not only are they expensive, but, in my view as a holistic health practitioner, most have negative side effects that can lead to a long, slow, ugly decline into medical disability, then death. Drugs seem almost universally toxic. They are hard on your liver and kidneys. They lead to other imbalances and other drug dependencies. I really didn't want to go down that path with my body. I was too well-trained, educated and experienced, and had too many natural and holistic therapies available to me to think that the pulmonologist was even a small part of the real answer. I went back to my natural healers. I went back to NAET and I booked myself a few sessions of craniosacral therapy. In one of these craniosacral therapy sessions, the therapist told me to visualize my lungs and tell my cells they really did not have to panic. Within a day or two of that session, all of the phlegm or, as I call it, "gunk" that customarily sat in the bottom of my lungs was gone. I was amazed. Then I knew. Just as I told all my clients and experienced from a therapist's point of view, my own body could be truly responsive to the right support. The soft tissue has the ability to heal in ways the medical community would not even consider; ways that would be called, to them, miraculous.

I also did yoga for lung health. I worked with homeopathic remedies, nutritional support and herbs. Though each treatment was not a cure by itself, they all contributed to a path toward healthy lung function. By the time of my next visit with the pulmonologist three months later, I felt much better. The first thing they had me do was a pulmonary function test. I passed this test with flying colors. The pulmonologist looked at me with detached disbelief. He told me he thought he was going to put me on the next stage of asthma treatment medication and it was not necessary now. He did ask me what I did to heal my lungs. I briefly told him but he dismissed it, and reluctantly told me to come back if I needed him.

Have you done anything since then to maintain your health in this regard?

Since then, it has been a matter of cat avoidance, getting booster treatments of NAET and maintaining a healthy lifestyle. I have used my inhaler twice in the last year, usually before or after I go to someone's house that has a cat. If I know beforehand, I will also take an antihistamine. I think that at some time I might try acupuncture as well, but haven't found the right practitioner yet.

What do you mean by typical Western medicine being the "long decline?"

I am going to get on my holistic high horse here; you will have to forgive me. I understand that the emergency room and some drugs save our lives and are necessary and many doctors do their best within a restrictive medical protocol. But as a consumer I have to think, "Why are they prescribing this drug? What is it really treating? What are the side effects, both short term and long term? What road am I going down with this treatment?" And, most important, "What are the best options for me to find a sensible, cost-effective, healthy, holistic and optimal cure?"

Another thing to keep in mind is the motivation of the doctors, therapists and the treatments. Most medical treatments involve drugs in one form or another. The drug companies have large, well-funded and effective marketing departments. They are more motivated by profit margins than successful treatment results. So then I ask myself, "What will make the drug companies the most money?" The common sense answer is: people who are chronically ill, dependent on multiple medications and, preferably, irreversibly addicted. There is no profit in fast and complete cures. There is profit in treating symptoms without curing them, and if the treatment results in other imbalances, which require further medication, all the better. The pill boxes get bigger and bigger, and the patient's livers, kidneys and bank accounts are increasingly burdened. I certainly agree that there are a good number of great life-saving medications, lots of scientists that truly want to create real solutions to our health struggles, and hopefully a good number of doctors that truly care about their patients.

Other things I keep in mind are the constraints that the insurance companies put on the kind of care I receive. The doctors are frequently treating based on the "standards of care" and protocols that the insurance companies dictate and will pay for. So who really is deciding what kind of health care I get? Is it the insurance company? They don't even know me. They just have a diagnosis code and a program that doesn't take into account so many aspects of my whole clinical picture. I am not surprised that the vast majority of the successful treatments that I use for my asthma are not covered by insurance. I pay cash. And I have done quite well with my health care, even though the times I have actually had health insurance in my life have been limited and sporadic. Therefore, I have been personally very motivated, by my pocketbook and by my pride, in my holistic healthcare education and experience, to find inexpensive, real, holistic and lasting cures to all my health challenges.

It is about business and profit margins. It is not about your health.

When I look at the medical industry, especially living where I do, surrounded by big pharmaceutical companies, this is what comes to my mind first: Are the doctors really trying to help me? Do they have my best interests in the forefront of their minds? Or are they hog-tied by a large, bureaucratic and profit-motivated industry that squeezes them down a very narrow lane each time they try to help someone? The pulmonologist I went to, despite the best qualifications, never said anything about a cure for my asthma. His assumption was a long and increasingly intensive course of treatment, hopefully leading to some kind of stabilization.

One thing I struggle with is where do you start in curing asthma? Is it diet, massage, NAET, craniocsacral therapy? What do you recommend asthmatics start with to cure themselves?

It depends. Does the person know what triggers the asthma? Do they know what the body is hyper-reacting to? Is it toxins or stressors in the environment? Food? There are so many things in food that people's bodies are overreacting to. It is finding out the specific thing that triggers you and then getting an overall wellness program. NAET is a good first step because it quickly and painlessly narrows down the list of allergic triggers for asthma. Then, treating the body with an overall holistic therapy that strengthens and balances is a necessary follow-up. Upledger's Craniosacral therapy is a wonderful technique, with some practitioners specializing in organ-function protocols. Other therapies, such as a variety of low-force chiropractic techniques or Eastern medicine — such as acupuncture or Ayurvedic medicine — would be good as well. I particularly like craniosacral therapy because, as a practitioner, I understand the power it has to balance and strengthen the whole body, as well as specific systems, in a way that's non-invasive, relaxing and effective.

Supplements and vitamins are also good. But it's best to find someone who is very knowledgeable about the ingredients, brands and treatment methods in order to have the best effect. If there is no one on hand, just go to a good health-food store or larger healthy market such as Whole Foods, and look at all the products and brands in the asthma and lung-health section. Which ingredients are the ones commonly used? Ask the store personnel which brands are best. Cheap vitamins and supplements can be useless. You may have to pay more money, but it's well worth it. The real test is, when you take the supplement or vitamin, do you notice a positive result? You should. If not, then go back and find another brand, product or consultant. For example, Standard Process is a trusted brand many chiropractors use, but is not widely available. With Standard Process, it is best to get a proper evaluation and diagnosis by the chiropractor and take the product they recommend.

Another approach is more geared toward mental empowerment and stress relief. It sounds crazy, but I use the power of my brain and intention every night to help me while I sleep. I have developed a short prayer protocol to ask my body and the universe for health and healing, even specific healing for my lungs. I have done this for years, and it helps a lot to take the edge off and get me by until my next therapy appointment. I'm sure doing this has helped to save me a lot of money by side-stepping many potential medical bills. The technique is described in my book, Magic Nights.

What about diet suggestions?

Along with eating as much healthy, whole, organic, raw and locally grown foods that you can, I would recommend limiting fatty dairy foods or anything that creates an excess of mucous production. But this must not be taken to excess. Mucous is absolutely necessary for many body functions, especially to protect the airways in the winter. "Good" fat is necessary for brain function. What you remove, you must replace. For example, I supplement my diet with a quality essential fatty-acids supplement, with heavy metals removed, as well as calcium citrate with magnesium in order to make up for decreasing my dairy intake.

Anything you would like to add?

I think people need to be aware of how much stress their body is under from our lifestyles and our environment. Asthma is just one of the ways the body overreacts to stress. There are all kinds of toxins and stressors all around us: from the fire retardants in our furniture to the artificial scents in our home products, to the electromagnetic pollution from our appliances and computers, to the drug remnants in our water supply, to the pesticides in our food, to the increasingly poor health created by our sedentary, yet 24/7 lifestyles.

Approach your asthma, as well as all your health challenges, from a place of self-empowered thinking. Think about all the sources of stress and allergic triggers and systematically and sensibly begin to find remedies that suit your lifestyle. The remedies don't have to be expensive — and remember how much it would cost to be chronically ill. Get educated about alternative therapies and remedies. Talk to friends for recommendations. Create for yourself a rounded and practical menu of good alternative practitioners and products that you like and trust. Believe in your power to work toward a true cure.

...

More about Dr. Hawn: www.MagicNightsBook.com.

Onward...

These 14 stories were collected to help David and the many Davids around the world. I hope these stories inspire asthmatics and the medical community to at begin to understand there are possibilities, outside of suffering needlessly, available.

As I continue to find more people who would like to share their stories on how they cured asthma, I will continue to add to this collection. It is my hope that with enough stories not only will more asthmatics' lives change, but perhaps it will encourage Western medicine to do the same. Of course, as Dr. Firshein said, there is not a cure for everyone. But I believe, in speaking with these people, that if there is not a cure for a particular individual, there is certainly a life to be had that includes significantly reduced consequences and symptoms of asthma.

I have never suffered from asthma, but I share the panic, stress and helplessness of the many who have had to watch those they love suffer. As is shown through these stories what triggers an individual's asthma and what cured it was unique to the individual. Some of these people were able to cure it with a single remedy on the first try.

David's journey to health has involved a bit of trial and error. He began his journey to finding a cure for asthma a little over seven months ago. The first six months yielded little except frustration and hundreds of euros in expenses. It was a visit to an acupuncturist who specialized in nutrition that changed David's life and asthma symptoms not only drastically but quickly.

The biggest change was he switched to a modified version of the Paleo diet, a diet consisting of lean proteins, fruits, vegetables, seafood, nuts and good fats. It took two weeks on this diet to see a remarkable improvement in his health. On first pass the diet seemed very restrictive. The good news is it is recommended he maintain this diet 80 percent of the time. Even his acupuncturist believes, "Everything in moderation including moderation."

Two weeks after David made the following dietary and lifestyle changes there was a remarkable improvement to his health:

- No sugar

- No wheat

- No dairy products (milk, cheese, yogurt etc)

- No soy

- No beans

- No refined or processed foods

- No alcohol

- No tomatoes

- No eggplant

- No potatoes

- No peppers

- No peanuts or peanut butter

- No fried foods

- No pasta

- No coffee

- Drinking room temperature water with meals

- No cooking in any oil except for coconut oil (vegetable broth and water are also good and less expensive options)

- Eating wild blue fish (tuna, salmon, anchovies, etc) multiple times per week

- Washing all sheets, blankets and pillows once a week

- Drinking a minimum of 2 liters (64 ounces of water) a day and more if possible

- Eating spelt bread in limited amounts (To note, David's acupuncturist believes it is better for him not to eat bread, but spelt bread is the best option for him if he is going to eat it.)

- Eating only organic meat

- Limiting his salt intake

- Drinking green tea

- Sporadic intake of vitamin C (typically 2000 milligrams at a time), magnesium (400 milligrams at a time) and spirulina.

- Working with an acupuncturist with significant educational training in nutrition who was also able to recommend supplements and dietary changes

- Taking specific supplements to aid with his digestion and overall well being as recommended by his acupuncturist.

David is not cured yet. However, he now requires his inhaler about the same number of times in a month that he would have used in one day prior to beginning the diet and changes noted above.

The last time I saw David use his inhaler was a few days ago. We were enjoying a friend's pool after surviving a day of extreme July temperatures. David was in the pool playing some impromptu version of one-on-one water polo with a friend. The physical exertion pushed David to reach for his inhaler as his friend, and follow competitor, waited.

Before, there were times when I would I see David use his inhaler and I would be sad for him. On this particular day I was hopeful: it had been days since I had seen David require his inhaler, and his competitor was a childhood friend who had decades prior cured himself of asthma.

...

About the Author

Linda Rubright is the founder of The Delicious Day (www.thedeliciousday.com), an online publication dedicating to profiling people who approach life, health and work in unconventional and inspirational ways.

If you have cured yourself of asthma or have significantly reduced your symptoms and would like to share your story, please contact linda@thedeliciousday.com.

Made in the USA
San Bernardino, CA
10 November 2016